THE
WIDOW
CHOSE RED?

My Journey with Jesus, John, and ALS

RACHEL KERR SCHNEIDER

The Widow Chose Red?
My Journey with Jesus, John, and ALS
Rachel Kerr Schneider

To contact the author: info@SpiritedProsperity.com

Edited and Published by

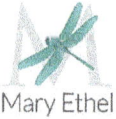

Mary Ethel

Mary Ethel Eckard
Frisco, Texas

Library of Congress Control Number: 2025908396
ISBN (Paperback): 978-1-966561-10-1
ISBN (Hardcover): 978-1-966561-11-8
ISBN (eBook): 978-1-966561-12-5

All scripture quotations, unless otherwise indicated, are taken from the Holy Bible, New International Version® NIV® Copyright © 1973, 1978, 1984, 2011 by Biblica, Inc.® All rights reserved.

DEDICATION

Dedicated to my husband John, because this
story wouldn't exist without him.
And to our sons, John III and Jake, through
whom the legacy of their father lives on.
Godspeed!
All my love... Live Your Dash....

ACKNOWLEDGMENTS

A shout-out to a few people who made this dream come true...

Erika and James, my parents, who instilled a belief in me
that I could do whatever I set my mind to.
They laid the foundation for my faith and still fortify me today.

Elaine, John's mom, who has been a
source of strength and resilience.

Lauri, the energizer bunny, who has had my back
and held the belief since the beginning.

Kevin, the unexpected bonus I never saw coming.
I'm still blindsided by his heart, spirit, and selfless nature
that has allowed me to be myself completely.

SPECIAL THANKS

Special thanks to Mary Anne, Jody, Sean, Elaine, James, Guy, Karen, Patty, Bill, Terry, and Kevin for previewing, reviewing, revising, advising, and sharing their thoughts as this manuscript morphed into the book you're holding today.

CONTENTS

SECTION IV: ALL THINGS NEW

FOREWORD

I've had the privilege of knowing Rachel Kerr Schneider for over a decade, and if there's one thing I've learned from her, it's that grace isn't just something she talks about, it's how she lives her life. Rachel has a quiet strength that's hard to describe but impossible to miss. Even when life dealt her the hardest blow imaginable, she walked through it with faith and dignity that inspired everyone around her.

This book is more than a story about loss, it's about love, faith, and resilience. Rachel doesn't shy away from the hard parts. She lets you into her moments of fear, sadness, and uncertainty—but what makes her story so powerful is how she responded. Even when the future felt unclear, she leaned on her faith and found strength she didn't know she had.

What strikes me most about Rachel's story is how gracefully she handled it all. She didn't try to be perfect or pretend to have all the answers—she simply trusted that God would carry her through. And He did. The moment when John asked, *"We don't have a choice, do we?"* could have been a breaking point. But Rachel met it with courage, love, and a quiet strength that defines who she is.

And here's the thing—Rachel didn't just show grace during that season of loss. She continues to live with that same grace today. She's a reminder that strength doesn't always look like having it all together. Sometimes it's just about showing up, trusting the process, and knowing that God is working even when you can't see it yet.

Rachel's story will stay with you long after you turn the last page. If you're facing your own hard season, I hope her story gives you comfort and strength. Remember, you don't have to have it all figured out. Just take the next step, lean on your faith, and trust that grace will meet you where you are.

Rachel, thank you for sharing your story with the world. Your strength, your faith, and your heart are a gift to everyone who knows you!

With love and gratitude,

Patty Aubery
New York Times Bestselling Author
Chicken Soup for the Christian Soul

INTRODUCTION

I have a saying over my mudroom doorway, "It's all good." It is a philosophy that has been preached to me and that I have talked about, used to instruct my boys, and applied to every situation. It may be in part based on Romans 8:28, *"For we know that all things work together for good to those who love God, to those who are called according to His purpose."* I believed it. I memorized it. I recited it to others. So how in the world was I supposed to rationalize it? Especially when we were about to embark on such a fateful journey.

John and I had been married for 21 years when everything changed. We had a marriage built on trust, respect, and faith. We enjoyed a relationship based on support and substance. We were blessed, we were a team who could tackle any challenge and function fabulously under pressure. We dealt with a lot, especially during his last three years.

When our life became an insurmountable challenge, I wondered if my faith was enough. I feared I wouldn't be able to handle the curveballs thrown at us. I had so many questions. How was I to keep living while someone I loved was dying? How could I make the dying process a "normal" part of living? I knew we had to give God total control of our lives and the situation, knowing those things didn't define us, and He would use them to refine us if we would surrender them to Him. But how were we to continue living with a diagnosis of death?

My faith did grow during this difficult season. I leaned

into God in the cloud of chaos and witnessed, in wonder and amazement, how He delivered me. I saw God's hand in the big and the small. I could see how He fortified my faith as I leaned on Him through the days, the diagnoses, and the decisions. That fortified faith was the glue that held me together mentally, physically, and spiritually. My heart was filled with gratitude for His power and presence, wisdom and strength, and I held on to His promise that with Him, all things are possible for those who believe. Gratitude was and is my way of life. Every day is a blessing, as we have no idea when our last day will be or what circumstances each day will bring.

It's time to tell the story of my life with John. In this book, I share the heartbreak and humor in supporting my husband during his terminal illness, giving insights into areas of life and death as discovered during the journey. The story is told to encourage those who are walking or have walked through a difficult season.

No matter where you are in your faith journey, the answer is always found in your relationship with God, Jesus, and the Holy Spirit. Knowing His word, goodness, grace, and mercy will carry you through whatever trial, tribulation, or struggle you may be facing. Seek every opportunity to fill your reservoir of faith so it is available for challenging times. Knowing who you are in Christ helps you to be better able to withstand any difficulty.

SECTION I
LIFE WITH JOHN

"For I know the plans I have for you," declares the Lord. "Plans to prosper you and not to harm you. Plans to give you hope and a future."

JEREMIAH 29:11

1

THE ARRANGED MARRIAGE

I met Elaine when I was an advertising rep for a trio of magazines in Dallas, Texas. She was the marketing and sales director for the first high-rise condo project in Dallas, the La Tour on McKinney Avenue. Her office was on one of the top floors, and I remember thinking, That's a very petite lady behind a very big desk in a very large office.

Was I a little intimidated? Maybe. Yet once she welcomed me and started chatting, the repertoire was easily established. I was in the middle of my pitch when she interrupted and asked, "Are you dating anybody?" I thought, well, that's a strange question to ask in the middle of a sales call. And although I was "seeing" someone long distance in Florida, I didn't miss a beat and said, "No." I was hoping this answer might help me score a few points in closing the deal. Her face lit up as she announced, "My son is moving to Dallas from Houston in a few days, and I would like to introduce you to him."

She then walked me over to the floor-to-ceiling windows and pointed down quite a few stories to a guy reclining in the sun next to the pool. "That's my other son, Ronald, who just graduated from SMU." I mentioned that I was a recent graduate as well and said, "I'd be happy to meet your other son anytime." I was secretly thinking, Oh, she will never remember and if she does, it may just move me closer to that sales agreement signature.

Elaine called me a few days later to invite me to a party at her home to welcome her son, John, to Dallas. This presented me with quite a dilemma. My parents were visiting that same weekend, and my cardinal rule was, when they're in town, don't go anywhere or do anything. Just hang out with them.

I couldn't take them to the party with me because I didn't know what would happen. I certainly wasn't going to leave myself exposed in that way. So, I cheated a little and said that I had a client event to attend. Since it was work-related, they had no issue. The day of the party arrived, and I headed over to Highland Park, the expensive side of town, not my usual stomping grounds. I was timely and figured I could get in and out in a relatively short period. How long could it take to say hello, exchange a few pleasantries, and exit stage right? The mission would be accomplished, and I could follow up on Monday to close the deal.

It was a nice warm evening in July and Elaine welcomed me with a big smile. She had set up a lovely area on her back deck, complete with a margarita machine. As she introduced me to her friends, she mentioned, "This is Rachel. She's the one that's here to meet John." That was a true statement, so I didn't let it get to me. One of her friends said, "Oh, Elaine, she's lovely. I'm sure John will like her."

Over an hour later, there was no sign of John. This was 1985. No cell phones, no texting, no John. Not impressed. Now, that got to me. Various reports insinuated that he was on his way, yet he wasn't showing up. By 10 p.m. I wasn't amused anymore, and I was set to depart the premises. At that moment, John's sister, Cheryl, let me know he was in the shower and would be down momentarily.

She then raced up the stairs to give him the 411 on me. I can just hear it now. He most likely asked, "What's she like?" And she probably responded, "A little hippy, and I'm not talking about as in 'peace out.' I'm talking in a childbearing type of way."

When John finally showed up, he was wearing a muscle shirt, shorts, and sunglasses at 10:30 p.m. because he didn't want me to see his bloodshot eyes. Not cool in my world. My opening line was, "Well, you're just lucky enough I waited around this long to meet you. Now I'm leaving." I might have been a little snarky in my delivery. Tone is an amazing tool, isn't it? John was taken aback, for sure.

I said a polite goodnight to Elaine. After all, my work here was done, and I headed out. John asked if he could walk me to my car. I said, "Sure, but if you think you're getting a kiss goodnight, you better think again, buddy." Again, he was caught off balance. I got to my car, said goodnight, nice to meet you, and he said the same.

I sped off into the night thinking, What a waste of an evening. But I carried out my commitment, still holding out hope of getting the deal done. You can imagine how surprised I was when I picked up the phone a few days later only to hear, "Hi, this is John Schneider. We met a few nights ago. I was hoping you would let me take you out on Friday night." I wanted to ask, "Are you nuts?" Instead, I took a breath. I happened to be free. So, I agreed.

When Friday arrived, John picked me up, still in his work

clothes, to which I remarked, "You have a job?" He grimaced and said, "Yeah, a pretty good one. Now can we go?" And believe it or not, he had a car too.

First Date | First Coming Out

Can you sense a little bit of hostility in my tone? I was definitely on an *"I don't need or want a man"* kick, so John was going to be fighting an uphill battle, at least on this date.

We headed to Lower Greenville Avenue, an area of town known for its trendy restaurants, hipster vibe, and eclectic music venues. We pulled into a dive of a spot called Aw Shucks, a hole in the wall known for its great oysters and seafood. John ordered raw oysters, which I love, and cold beers, which I don't. I'm not sure whether he was nervous but while setting the food on the roughhewn picnic table outside, a full cup of beer accidentally toppled on the table, the oysters, and me.

John couldn't apologize enough, and I couldn't have cared less. I could tell this wasn't going to end well, and I just wanted it to end. Yet, somehow, by the end of the night, I half-heartedly agreed to see him again, and that was how we began. After sharing the story with our sons many years later, they coined the term for our relationship: "an arranged marriage." That's how they saw it, given that Mama Lane (Elaine) set it all up. And I guess they weren't wrong.

During our beginning days of getting to know one another, I also started getting to know his younger brother, Ronald, who was my age. Irony of ironies, we were both at SMU at the same time: 1982-1984. I was in business school and wasn't sure where Ronald was, but suffice it to say, our paths never crossed on campus. But when I started dating John, Ronald and I saw more of each other, and getting to know him made me look at my deep religious beliefs.

Growing up in Jackson, Mississippi, my father was Southern Baptist and my mother was Lutheran. We spent Sunday morning in the Lutheran church on the front row with Mom, and Sunday evenings at Bible drill and Training Union at the Baptist church. In between was lunch and quiet time. I was taught that drinking alcohol, smoking, and dancing would land me in hell. Not that I believed "everything" I was told. Call me naïve, please, because even today, I have a trusting character and don't jump to conclusions unless they are obvious. Even then, it can take a while.

One day, Ronald invited me to happy hour at Uncle Julio's Mexican restaurant in Dallas. I got into his Mercedes, which was always covered with cassettes, his briefcase, file folders, and real estate listing information (he was

> And there I was. At the age of 22, I had my first bona fide interaction with a certified real gay person. And guess what? Lightning didn't strike either one of us.

a realtor). His car was his mobile office. He loved loud music, so he put in a cassette tape and turned up the volume. As we were zipping toward the restaurant, Ronald turned to me and blurted out, "You know I'm gay, right?"

I looked at him, driving with his sunglasses on, grinning from ear to ear, and replied in my typical naïve Southern girl drawl, "I wasn't sure." Isn't that the most politically correct answer possible? He answered, "Well, I just didn't want you to be wondering, and I knew that John probably wouldn't say anything because I hadn't come out and said it 'loud and proud' to him. He just knows."

And there I was. At the age of 22, I had my first bona fide

interaction with a certified real gay person. And guess what? Lightning didn't strike either one of us. Ronald didn't morph into a different person, and my feelings for or toward him didn't change. He was still the smart, witty, successful, fun, explosive, volatile guy that he always was. He knew how "religious" I was, so it was probably harder for him to share than I realized.

Road Trip to New Beginnings

John was promoted and his new position as regional office manager took him to Pennsylvania. It was during this time that we realized I wasn't going anywhere permanently without a ring on my finger, so we got engaged.

After that, my crossing paths with Ronald became a full-on intersection. Getting together with Ronald probably should have come with those crossing guard rails they have at railroads; the ones that make the driver stop so they don't attempt to cross the tracks without warning.

Ronald was always up for a good time, yet one never knew what might wreck that FAST! I never gave it much thought, because our relationship was based on mutual admiration. He adored me, and I was impressed with his knowledge, success, work ethic, dress code, and his ability to be spontaneous and have fun. Ronald was always there to lend support to us as we bounced around the country with relocations. He was our moving advocate, weighing in on subdivisions, school districts, commutes, and most importantly, resale values. He could walk into a house and give the 411 in ten seconds flat. He knew if a place needed too much work, or if it was the steal of a deal, with surprising speed and accuracy. For instance, he looked at over 40 homes on our behalf when we purchased our home in Flower Mound, Texas.

I knew he was genuinely a good person but seemed to be compensating for something. His relationship with John had its challenges, and I was a buffer that kept the sharp edges from getting too close. Both Ronald and John had an intense desire to succeed, which they both did early and often.

John was living in Philadelphia, working and settling in. He started attending a small Lutheran church in King of Prussia, PA. Pastor Greg and his wife, Idalynn, were a young dynamic spirit-filled couple with a young son. Greg was especially effective in connecting and communicating. We started planning our wedding, and John considered flying Pastor Greg in for our ceremony, but since our budget was so tight (we were footing the bill) that didn't happen. But it speaks volumes to how much John thought of him. It was the beginning of a relationship that has remained significant, special, and sacred to this day.

Because John was destined to climb the corporate ladder, I decided before we were married that John's career would come first, and I would personify the "trailing spouse syndrome." Our plans were to get married in Dallas and then I would move to Philadelphia.

In preparation for the move, I boxed and shipped most of my possessions to Philly, including my desk and bedroom furniture, which was antique style and purchased by my mom. We didn't have a lot of money to pay for moving, so most of my furniture stayed with Nicole, my sister, who planned to stay in the townhome that my parents had purchased.

The plan was to road trip in my white Cutlass Supreme, a car I loved. My father had purchased it from Steel City Olds in Birmingham, Alabama. Rumor had it that the car was meant to be given to Miss Alabama, but maybe she didn't want it. It was a gorgeous car. John hated it, but it was what we were taking to Philadelphia.

I took the car into the shop to have it looked over before we made the 1,500-mile road trip. They found something that needed to be addressed, and then something else, and they were still working on it the day before our wedding. John was out of his mind worried that we would not have a car to drive. The car repairs totaled about $1,000, which we were not prepared for, but we managed to scrape the money together. We were young, didn't have money, and our parents didn't have any to give us. We were on our own and I wasn't working yet. We were also paying for our wedding and now the car repairs. Luckily, John had that good job, remember?

We were married in Dallas in September 1987, which was a lovely affair with 125 people. At our reception, which was held at the Bonaventure, we had hot and cold hors d'oeuvres and a cake, along with champagne and beer. Ronald was a member of the Crescent Club located on the top floor of the Crescent building. He hosted an after-party after our reception and several people went. John and I didn't go because we didn't know anything about it. It must have been quite the bash because my youngest brother, Sean, ended up with alcohol poisoning and was too sick to fly home. He had to take the bus back to Louisiana.

We spent our wedding night at the Four Seasons Hotel in Las Colinas, Texas. The suite was lovely even though my friends, Ki and Pat and their husbands, John and Rex, snuck in and posted all kinds of fun words over the bed, left us a bottle of champagne, and put paper everywhere. Not just any paper. I had worked on a fundraiser for the Wadley Guild for a few years. My job was to help with the graphic design and create the program for the event. It was a big deal and a big program with professional portraits of over a hundred society women. The paper that my friends used to "redecorate" the suite was that program.

The next morning, we headed to Elaine's house to have brunch with her and her relatives. When we got to the car, we were surprised to see they had also gotten those keys and stuffed so much paper into it that we couldn't get in. It was hilarious.

After brunch, we started our trip to Philadelphia with a planned overnight stay in Nashville, the halfway point. We didn't have cell phones or GPS in those days, but we had a map and interstate signs pointing us to Nashville. We arrived around 8:30 p.m., but we didn't know exactly where we were. Were we on the outskirts? Were we in a bad section? John pulled into some "no-tell" motel in a seedy area of town. He parked the car under a light to lessen the chances of somebody breaking in. We were probably just a couple of blocks from being in a nice part of town, but John wouldn't ask; that's not the way he rolled. The next morning, we finished the drive to King of Prussia, PA, which is about 20 miles northwest of Philadelphia. Prussia rhymes with Russia and for this southern gal, it might as well have been a foreign country. (We did eventually take our honeymoon four years later to the Grand Lido in Jamaica. We had a lovely time!)

Philadelphia

It isn't that far-fetched, is it? John and I met in July 1985 and by September 1987, we were husband and wife, driving to our new home in my just had to be repaired to the tune of one thousand dollars white T-top Cutlass Supreme. What a perfect way to begin our life together, a mega-hour-day road trip in a questionable car.

We drove up to the two-bedroom condo John had purchased. We had my things and the few pieces of furniture I shipped.

Everything else was hand-me-downs from his mom. We were grateful.

On my birthday, just one month after arriving in Philly, I woke up to find a new four-door, black Honda Accord in the driveway. I guess John realized my car wasn't going to be a good match for the weather or driving conditions in our new locale. So, he sold my car and picked out another one for me. I had nothing to do with it, that's just what I got, and I was happy.

What a perfect way to begin our life together, a mega-hour-day road trip in a questionable car.

Same story with the first two cars I drove. My dad got me a lime green Vega, rusted out around the windshield and the floorboards. He paid $800 for it. I learned how to drive in it and drove it all around my hometown of Jackson, MS for a while. I was thankful. Months later, my younger brother Sean came running into the house yelling, "There's a midget outside; there's a midget outside." I said, "Sean, you cannot run around yelling 'There's a midget outside.' You know, people have feelings and I'm sure that person is hurt by your words. That's not a very nice thing to yell." He looked at me and said, "Come here, come here. I'll take you to see the midget."

He led me outside to an MG Midget sitting in the driveway. I didn't know a car could be so small. Dad had gotten the car from a gentleman whose son had one too many traffic tickets, so his dad took the car away and my dad bought it for me. The problem was, I didn't know how to drive a stick.

What a picture it was to see Dad teaching me. He's a big man, 6 foot + with a large frame, jammed into that tiny MG, and I don't know how long it had been since he had driven a stick. It was a rocky road for a while. But that car got me through my junior and senior years of high school. I put it into so many tight spaces that sometimes the only way I could get out was to unsnap the top and crawl out. What a picture I was, with my big hairspray hair, dressed to the nines, wiggling out of that canvas roof.

Now, as a newly married woman living in Philadelphia, I was the owner of a new Honda Accord. It's interesting because, years later, when we were moving to Minnesota, John sent me to the Acura dealership saying, "Go get an MDX." I answered, "Okay, I'll go get an MDX. But before I do, there are two things I need to know. One. If I run off the road, will I be able to get out of a snowbank? And two, will the kids have an entertainment system so if we are sitting in a snowbank and waiting for someone to come and pull us out, they will be occupied?" While I can drive anything in a pinch, all these years later, I'm still driving an MDX. His suggestion was a good one. I love everything about them.

Adjusting to Married Life

There were a lot of adjustments that took place that first year. When John and I were married, it was just the two of us. We didn't live next to our parents or family. We were on our own, which was great, and we would figure everything else out day by day. That's a strong testimony of our upbringing and our confidence and ability to rely on each other and ourselves. We've always known that we had the support of our family, but we didn't need them next door, in the same state, in the same country, or on the same continent.

But being in a new city with no friends, no contacts, and no internet was no fun. John went to work while I stayed home looking for a job. He was climbing the corporate ladder while I was trying to find my place with an ad agency. Before marriage, I had my own advertising and public relations company. I spent my days developing brochures, events, and radio commercials, for clients including the Staubach Company and Sullivan Development. I worked with a great team: Bob, his wife Catherine, and Barbara, who took direction and produced great material. Letting go of that business was difficult, and I'm not sure John understood what it took to walk away from it.

I eventually landed a position as an account executive with a real estate-based advertising agency in downtown Philly. They thought I was a great representation of Delta Burke from *Designing Women*. Big hair, southern drawl, and mounds of makeup. You get the picture.

The president and founder of the company was Richard. He lived on the Main Line which is an affluent area outside Philadelphia. He also owned the four-story building where the agency was located. He spoke at conferences, developer's conventions, and industry events. Most of the focus was on custom-built, single-family homes. People would hear him at these conferences and then hire the agency.

> They thought I was a great representation of Delta Burke from *Designing Women*. Big hair, southern drawl, and mounds of makeup.

My boss, an account supervisor, was a "mad" Russian guy named Alex. Jay was the other account supervisor. He was a young guy who favored himself as a protégé to Richard because they were both Jewish.

For an old-school ad agency, we were cutting edge. The first floor was reception, the second floor was media buying and copywriting, and the third floor was account execs, account supervisors, and Richard's office. The fourth floor was creative and typesetting.

I worked with Alex and Jay. The account executives were the liaison between the creative team at the agency and the client. The team consisted of me; Todd, who was a nice, kind, and funny blonde guy; Tricia, another blonde, who was a space case; and Perry, aka *God's gift to advertising*, who fancied herself as an account supervisor, but wasn't. She had gone to some Ivy League school, I think, or that was the impression she gave. Though I wasn't aware of it at the time, she and I were competing. We were a melting pot of personalities and egos. During the time I worked there, more than a few clashes were happening on the third floor.

As an account executive, I was assigned the clients I was to work with. I knew the importance of personality and being able to relate to different kinds of people. I excelled at it. Richard decided who would work with which account based on temperament and personality. We were also assigned a creative team, an art director, and a copywriter. Teams were always changing, so we worked with everybody, almost all the time. Because everything had to be scheduled, we worked with Lynn, who was in charge of traffic. She was in control of how soon a project could be done or whether it would meet deadlines. I learned quickly that it was a wise career move to get along with Lynn.

Our job was to meet with the client, find out what they wanted, determine what they needed, pitch the idea, and work with the art director to bring the idea to life. The creative and typesetting guys on the fourth floor did not meet with the client, and if they were ever asked to, they would go into a panic.

There was a lot of handholding with the clients. We had to keep track of our hours, how much time we spent on the phone with a client, and every time we had a meeting. We did a lot of newspaper advertising: we would develop a campaign, and it would run for one to three months. We would coordinate special events for clients including grand openings, and press events.

Most of our customers were located on the East Coast, although we did have one client in Chicago. Some of my co-workers and I were commissioned to travel by air to meet the client, see the site, see the product, and develop a plan. I didn't know it at that time, but it was unusual for all of us to travel by air, so I'm not sure if the purpose was to decide who would handle the account or whether they would split up parts to various people. We got the account, which was good since the flight home was not good. Practically from takeoff to landing, we bounced around like kernels of popcorn being popped. After that, no one wanted to leave Philadelphia.

Another account was with the Silver Companies. Carl was the founder, and he had one son, Larry, who was the heir apparent. They were a multi-faceted business with commercial, residential, multi-family, senior, hotel, and construction properties. They needed a corporate brochure, so we proposed producing one featuring the different categories and including the men who ran each division. There were multiple components to the brochures, and it was a big assignment. At the time, I was 25 years old and didn't get the respect I should have because I was a woman, and they assumed I didn't know what I was doing.

Ray was the art director in charge of the creative for the Silver Companies, including brochures, ads, etc. He was difficult to work with and moody. I don't think he had done a corporate brochure before, and it was a huge undertaking, especially for a company that wasn't clear what they wanted. But we pushed forward. We opened a file for the development of the brochure, Lynn put us on the schedule, and Ray had three to four days to put together an initial concept.

After the concept design, I would take it to the client to get approval and then we would lay it out and schedule copy, photography, and interior layout. For photography, I would round up all assets needed and schedule locations to take the pictures. Then I would meet with the client's staff to get their approval of the photos and the text they wanted to use for that part of the brochure. There was a lot to do, a lot of balls in the air at the same time, and a lot of scheduling both with the client and inside the agency. Once the brochure was produced, they were pleased with it, which was a big feather in my cap, so to speak.

Would you believe that the same brochure was used many years later as an introduction to a date? Here's the Reader's Digest version of that story.

Enter Deborah Berman. I knew her as Debbie, both of us were members of a teen modeling board for a large regional department store, Gayfers. Hence the Gayfer Girls (GGs). We attended rival high schools, competed in the Jackson Jr. Miss Pageant, graduated high school, and went our separate ways. No big deal, right? It happens all the time.

While I was doing research on the GGs for an upcoming reunion, I came across Debbie's wedding announcement in the local Jackson newspaper. I did a double-take when I saw that she wed a man named Larry Silver. One thing led to another and, by the time I was done with the rabbit trail, I realized that, yes indeed, it was in fact the same Larry Silver that I had worked for.

So, on my next visit to West Palm Beach, Florida, I reached out to Debbie via social media. I attended her concert, and we ended up having dinner together. You can imagine Larry's surprise when I reminded him about the brochure and began to ask about some of the guys who worked with him. Debbie looked at me and asked,

"You did THAT brochure?" I replied, "Yes I did, and it was some kind of project."

She went on to share that back in the day, before cell phones, Google, etc., a mutual friend suggested she meet Larry. When she asked Larry for a photo, he sent her the corporate brochure which featured a great photo of him and his father, front and center. Who knew? God knew! I love it when He surprises us in such fun and fabulous ways.

One of my first friends in Philadelphia was Emily, who was a copywriter. We would take our lunch break together whenever we could and would often walk outside. Emily opened my eyes to quite a few things. She was a great reprieve from the tension of personalities I had to deal with during the workday. She introduced me to sub sandwiches, which I loved, and falafel from a truck, which I didn't.

I learned that in big urban areas, pigeons are everywhere. And before I knew it, a pigeon pooped on top of my head. I've heard it is good luck. REALLY? I was mortified. I had big hairspray hair. I couldn't just rinse it out! So, I stepped into McDonalds, found the bathroom, and worked on getting the white poop out of my hairspray hair while trying not to mess up my entire head. Emily was cracking up. I thought she was going to wet her pants. Me? Not so much.

I wish I could say that things got better after the pigeon poop incident, but they didn't. It seemed that adjusting was becoming my way of life, requiring more resilience with each passing day, and I was struggling to keep getting back up.

CHAPTER

2

MORE TRANSITIONS

Pennsylvania

Downtown Philadelphia was not my favorite place. I had never worked in a big city, I wasn't used to tall buildings, and I didn't like not being able to see the sun. In Dallas, the sun is visible, even downtown. It was unnerving and somewhat depressing. That city and I were not friends.

Then, as I was adjusting to being in this depressing new place, John was put into the Peterbilt training program which meant he had to stay in Dallas for three months. He would work in the factory; some weeks in the paint booth, some weeks in welding, and other weeks he would be on the line. He loved it.

But not me. I was stuck in the condo on my own. During this timeframe, I suffered a lot from migraines, which was traumatic. The pain would cause me to lose entire weekends. I was left alone in Philly, and it wasn't pretty. Pastor Greg and the Lutheran church were a great blessing during that time. When John was home, we attended church together and were involved in several of the young couple's events. When John was away, I attended by myself. It was a place of community and gave me comfort. It made me feel less alone.

After John completed his training program in Dallas, he was sent to Seattle to further his training with Peterbilt Parts and Service. The cross-country commute was not cost-effective, so I relocated to Seattle to live with John in a corporate apartment. Again, I struggled with no sense of direction. I wondered what having a job or career might look like since John was moving around in this program. I felt lonely, stuck, confused, and lost. It was at this time I sought out my first therapist, Susan. I didn't tell anyone except John. I knew asking for help carried the stigma that strong people should be able to overcome stuff on their own; only weak people needed help. Sound familiar?

Susan was considerate, calm, and easy to work with. She helped me realize that John was not to blame. I had willingly and lovingly decided to be his wife and support his career. It was a gift from my heart I had given to him. It was time to stop holding him hostage and to investigate what would bring me joy for the next three months. I took golf lessons and cooking lessons. We bought mountain bikes, hiked Mount Rainier, took weekend trips, and visited his alma mater, Lewis and Clark, in Portland.

After three months in Seattle, John was sent to Fremont, California, a city just outside of San Francisco, to begin his next phase of training. As we were packing to drive down, news flashed of the earthquake happening during the World Series. Bridges were down and buildings were on fire. "John, are you sure it's a good time to move to California?" He replied, "Everything will be fine." We drove to Fremont, moved into an apartment, and within a few days, John went back to work.

San Francisco

Our living quarters in Fremont were not in the best section of town, but at least we were about a forty-minute drive from John's father and his second wife, Trish. We spent Christmas with them while we lived so close. We made the holiday about the experience of preparing a meal. It was the first time I made lobster bisque, which was delicious but exhausting. The holiday was wonderful, and I set a gorgeous table. I was grateful we had family so close by.

Other than that, I didn't know anyone, and I fell into a depression. John would come home from work, and I would still be in my pajamas. He didn't know how to help me, but he was good about not making it worse. Maybe because he sensed it was temporary. I felt like it was forever. I knew I needed to find a job, but I had no idea where we would be living after John finished his training, and commuting in California can be an all-out cluster.

In my job search, I attended a networking/career counseling center a few times a week to use the computer and look through postings. My first opportunity was a part-time job doing the marketing for the parks and recreation division of the City of Milpitas. I was responsible for marketing events and creating a character campaign for the department. I soon realized I was spending more hours than part-time, so I started searching again.

Looking through ads in the newspaper, I somehow snagged an interview with an agency in the city, Channels, run by a woman named Leslie. She seemed bright, assertive, fashionable, and successful. Her agency was small and had a staff of three people, and we all worked in the same office. No cubicles; just one big open space. No privacy, no personal space, and no idea how difficult it would be. I commuted to the city every day, 45 minutes each way, and paid for parking. It wasn't all bad, but it didn't take too long to realize the work environment wasn't a good fit, so I started searching again.

By this time, John had completed his training program, and we had purchased a small duet home in Danville. He carpooled with two guys in the morning and was adapting to his new position.

My newspaper sessions yielded a new position as a marketing associate with Baron Data, a company that developed a software program for court reporters. I was interviewed by Rick Savage and Diane Galvin. She was sharp and smart, and I was excited to work with her. A week after I was hired, she gave her two-week notice and told me I would be working for Rick, her boss. Within months, Baron Data was acquired by Stenograph Corporation, based in Chicago, so we had to create a new product line that represented the merged company. I was new to the industry and new to the company which was now part of another company.

After a while, Rick hired Melissa to help with marketing, and then he left to take a position as Vice President of Sales and Marketing with Triad Systems, located in Livermore, California. Triad Systems was the largest supplier of data to the automotive aftermarket, which was how car parts were searched, ordered, and distributed to service dealers all over the country. This was before the internet, so CDs were sent to the dealers, and updates were sent monthly. They also had divisions that dealt with hardware and data for both industries and customer support.

It was a big company with a huge campus. Rick reported to Shane and wanted me to work with him doing marketing, advertising, trade shows, media, collateral materials, sales meetings, etc. As I walked across the giant campus to meet with

Shane, I didn't feel I had a background in tech, but I did have a good background in marketing, scheduling, working with vendors, and buying media. Rick wanted me there despite my lack of experience in the tech world. Shane interviewed and hired me. He was in charge of almost everything, and I would report to him.

I was the only woman working in this position at this time. Ken trained me; he was also the person I was replacing. He did not like me at all. As I shadowed him to learn the job, he told me he was going back into the field, which is what he wanted to do, but he wasn't getting the territory he wanted. As in a lot of companies, great field salespeople are brought in-house and put in charge of different areas: sales and marketing, or whatever. But the reason people go into sales is to be out in the field, to do things on their own, to enjoy independence, and not have to report to anyone except their sales manager. And as long as they're making their numbers, everyone leaves them alone, for the most part.

When I was 30, I was awarded a trip for two to St. John, US Virgin Islands. The division awarded the trip to someone not in the field that they believed had the most impact in supporting the sales representatives and helping them achieve their goals. I didn't realize how big a deal it was because I had never worked for a company that large. My resilience was paying off.

Then, change hit again. Peterbilt was closing its California location and employees were given the option for relocation to Dallas. They were flown to DFW with their spouses for a weekend tour of the office and the area. Many people chose not to relocate. Having spent time in California, they found Dallas to be "ugly, full of concrete, glass, and metal with no natural beauty." We were happy to leave the overpriced lifestyle of California, mindful that the cost of living in Dallas would be different.

When I told Rick we were moving to Dallas, he said, "You're

not quitting this job. You can just do it from there. You can spend two weeks here and two weeks there." He was ahead of his time. This was before telecommuting was a thing, but he was used to having the sales reps come in and do training. They would be in the office for a week and then go back into the field. I had a telephone and a computer, and there was an Extended Stay hotel close to the office, so that's what I did.

Dallas, Texas

John and I found and bought a house in Plano, a suburb north of Dallas, thanks to help from his brother, Ronald, who was excited to have us back in Texas. He coordinated the updates for us before we arrived.

We were lucky to have great neighbors on either side. They couldn't figure out why John had more furniture than a single guy needed, or why there was a woman who could come in for a week and then be gone the next.

We set up my office on the first floor and I commuted between Dallas and California until I got tired and wanted to spend more time at home. I talked with Rick about my decision, and we parted on good terms. He was more comfortable having someone else fill my role, which was a relief.

I knew I needed to get back to work so when a friend, Susan, approached me and told me about working with Partylite, and developing new markets, my answer was an immediate YES! I had experience in all of these things, and I knew that with hard work and great sales, I could become the first regional vice president in Dallas and put Dallas on the map for the company. All I needed to do was find six women to grow groups of at least six that would sell X amount per month at the same time and BOOM! I would make dollars off my own sales, team sales, and organizational sales.

I started selling candles and home décor with Partylite and I approached it like any other sales job. I networked, attended chamber meetings, placed ads, and advertorials, handed out samples everywhere I went, and booked shows, sponsored new women, promoted leaders, and held training workshops and special events. Susan was also my boss. We had a call every Monday to review sales, sponsoring, promotions, and the calendar, just like I did in my advertising days. Except this wasn't a corporate gig. I was an independent rep with a mission.

John was fine with me working so much because he was just as busy. Climbing the corporate ladder can take all someone has to give. John's commute to Denton was 45 minutes and he was always early, so his days were long. If I had a Partylite show, I would usually miss him because I would leave early to avoid rush hour traffic.

One of the best perks of working with Partylite was the friends I made while involved. Kara was one of the first consultants I sponsored, and she quickly became a regional vice president in Texas. Paula was the assistant to Kara, and she was also a Partylite leader. A native of Lancaster, Pennsylvania who relocated to Texas on a basketball scholarship to the University of Texas, Paula was a ton of fun and became one of my closest friends. We became closer than sisters.

As my business grew, Paula's role within our family grew as well. She continued with her Partylite business, but she would also come to our house and help me manage my business and the boys. We spent a lot of time together.

When John took the position to run Larson Companies, an executive assistant position did not exist, and Paula had become such a part of our family that John negotiated a spot for her. She became his work-wife and continued to be my closest friend.

Paula was born on July 4th, so one year I threw her a surprise 40th birthday party at Casa Grande, Elaine's house in Palm Desert. She was part of a big Catholic family, so when her sisters and mother came, combined with our friends from Dallas, Weesie, Cheri, Jennifer, and Tami, it was a lively crowd. That party was probably one of the best things we ever did, so good in fact that it morphed into an annual girls' trip for many years. We enjoyed laying in the sun all day, making our own dinner, and going to the casino or the outlet mall in Cabazon. We would play cards, read books, swim, or watch movies. These were wonderful moments that helped us build remarkable relationships and friendships.

An Unexpected Diagnosis

We took a vacation to Hawaii with John's sister, Cheryl, and her husband Tom. Ronald brought his partner, Darren. The six of us had a great visit. We hiked, swam, shopped, ate, and drank our way through a few relaxing days.

I was a Barbara Walters fan, so while there, we watched a program where she was interviewing Greg Louganis, the 1984/1988 Olympic gold medalist. He wanted to let the world know that he was gay and had been diagnosed with HIV. After we returned home, we learned that Ronald was planning on telling us about his diagnosis while in Hawaii but lost his nerve. He contracted it from someone while at SMU but had only recently been diagnosed, and he was involved with an experimental drug program at Baylor and was managing to stay relatively well.

This was 1995 and the world was just beginning to understand the connection between HIV and AIDS. People were paying attention primarily because a diagnosis usually meant death, a painful and ugly one at that. I was aware but not paying attention. It didn't affect me personally, and I had more important things to focus on, or so I thought. And I only knew one gay person at that time, so what were the chances I would ever have to be concerned with AIDS?

> I only knew one gay person at that time, so what were the chances I would ever have to be concerned with AIDS?

Ronald didn't allow his diagnosis to get in the way of work until it did. He was diagnosed at a young age with a disease for which there was no cure. So, he opted for experimental treatments. John and I had the privilege of being on the journey with him, full of promise, pondering, pit stops, and pain, but also full of joy, laughter, and life-changing moments that still speak to my soul today.

John and I were humming along just fine, and John was promoted to region manager, the youngest one ever. This promotion involved a move to Chicago. I hated leaving Dallas, but I had some news of my own to share with John.

Another New Beginning

It was 1996. We had been married for almost 10 years and endured countless questions, "When are you going to have a baby?" Instead of having a baby, when John turned 30, I had a surprise party for him. The biggest surprise? We got a dog, an Airedale to be exact, and we named her Trixi. I would have much rather had a baby at this point, but the birthday party was great, and Trixi turned out to be a pretty good dog. Airedales by nature are a bit high-strung, which is why she did so well with John. I, on the other hand, helped her mellow out a little bit. I'd like to think I had the same impact on John, but it usually took a few drinks to loosen him up.

I was 34 when I got pregnant. John was thrilled. I was cautiously optimistic as I joked, "I just got screwed by the newest region manager." Crude but true.

We were in Naperville, Illinois, a suburb of Chicago, looking at houses, and I was cranky, tired, and stifling morning sickness. Our real estate agent, Mary, was terrific. We found a big house situated on a cul-de-sac with a basement, and a big backyard overlooking a retaining pond in the community of Oakhurst. Ronald came into town and gave his blessing for our new home. Of course, we were headed right into winter, which is one of the bleakest times of the year. That's the thing about living in the Chicago area. In the winter, it doesn't give a lot of sun. It stays cloudy and cold, with lots of snow.

We were busy getting the house ready and I was on my own for that. So, it was not the best of times, but it most certainly wasn't the worst of times.

Jeanie, my good friend from Texas, came and helped do a mural on the wall for the nursery. The painting was of clouds with soft blues and pale yellows in a gender-neutral décor since we didn't know whether we were having a boy or a girl.

We picked out a name for a female – Erika Elaine, after my mom and John's mom. I thought that name sounded cool. And, of course, since we come from that southern tradition of that generational thing, if it was a boy, we would name him John William Edward Schneider, III. After all, we had a John Sr. and we had a John, Jr., so a III was the logical next step for our son.

I found a female ob/gyn that I liked, which was great since I didn't like being pregnant. I put my best foot forward by getting the cutest maternity clothes I could find. Always the fashionista.

John was traveling a lot. I was restarting my Partylite business. I had left a very successful team in Dallas and would now have to recreate that success in my new city. The company had a policy called "adoption" wherein someone like me who did not have a leader in the area could be trained by another regional vice president. I chose to go with Kay, a virtual celebrity in the world of Partylite. She was a Senior Regional Vice President and multiple award winner at every conference. I wanted to be just like her.

My team in Texas was growing, yet I knew if I could access the keys to Kay's kingdom, we would all be sailing on the sea of success very soon. I would download everything to the Texas leader team, and the information was instrumental in their rapid growth and promotion of three regional vice presidents, all in my organization. Kay was a brilliant trainer, but her leadership skills were a bit militaristic, and she could be especially harsh. I remember making the one-hour drive to her home for a leader meeting only to be locked out because we were 15 minutes late. This was before cell phones, GPS, and texting.

I attended the regional Christmas party and met another pregnant woman about my age, Denise, due around the same time. This was her fourth child and my first. Her family was from Louisiana, so we had the southern thing in common, and she became one of my dearest friends. I'm not sure how because we didn't live near one another, but we managed to bond during training, workshops, regional meetings, conferences, and all the travel time in the car.

During this time, John and I realized we needed to find a church home. Relocating and finding a new church was just one of the patterns of our life together. We found a church, Good Shepherd, that seemed like it might work. We attended the service, listened to the pastor, and decided we would come back. As we were leaving the narthex area, I noticed a wall with photographs of their pastors on it. Suddenly I saw someone who looked familiar. I looked at John and said, "Hey, that's Pastor Greg. It looks like he might be a pastor here." John looked at me and said, "Rachel, we just sat through the service. That wasn't him."

I answered, "Well, I think if I read the bulletin correctly, this guy was filling in. Maybe Pastor Greg is on vacation." John smirked and said, "No. I think you're reading the whole thing wrong." So, I replied, "Well, let's come back next week and take a look." John agreed, though I'm sure the whole time he was thinking to himself that my pregnancy hormones were kicking in and had gotten the best of me.

We went back the next week. As the service began, we saw the pastor and, as he was delivering the sermon, I elbowed John intensely. He looked at me like I was a crazy woman. I could tell a couple of times that the pastor would look at us and hesitate, only because he wasn't sure he knew us. I can only imagine a pastor looking into a sea of faces every week, getting familiar with his flock, and knowing their seating preferences. New faces could cause confusion.

At the end of the service, as the pastor was greeting everyone leaving the sanctuary, John and I hung back. We knew we would need more time than a normal, "A good sermon, thank you for your words, or good to see you." I was so excited I could hardly contain myself. By the time we got to Pastor Greg, he looked at us and said, "I think I know you guys." I said, "Of course you do. We're Rachel and John Schneider. We knew you back in King of Prussia, Pennsylvania." He looked at John and said, "You're with the truck company, right?" John answered, "Yes, I am." Pastor Greg said, "Well, I was looking at you guys and then I got this awful feeling. Oh no, I don't mean awful. I mean I got this feeling that maybe I knew you. What are you doing here?" I answered, "Well, John got promoted and now we're living here, and we're expecting a baby."

Having the connection with Pastor Greg was nothing less than Divine Intervention. My time in Chicago was one of the more difficult phases of my life. Part of it might have been postpartum, but it was a difficult time in our marriage; nonetheless.

I dare say that my Partylite business saved me in some ways because it offered me a connection with other women, but it was still hard. I had to find babysitters to watch the boys when I had shows. I had to coordinate my time on the phone to book shows, talk to my team, do training, etc. John and I, more often than not, were like ships passing in the night. I know as I say this that I'm not the only young wife and mother who has experienced this in her marriage.

It was at this time that I, for the first time, considered life without John as my husband. I was desperate to get his attention to realize the seriousness of the situation. I said, "John, I'm not happy. I'm not feeling the love." His answer mirrored mine. He said, "I'm not feeling it either, but we don't have a choice, do we?" I answered, "I think we do."

At that time, my parents were living in Australia, and I called them and spoke with my father, not my mother. I told him that I was considering a possible separation. In his calm way, he talked me off the ledge. He didn't get emotional; he just kept it factual, although he heard me and acknowledged how I was feeling. He also reminded me of the vows I had taken and the covenant I made. This wasn't just between me and John; it was me and John and Jesus. His reminder was fortifying for me. It didn't make the situation instantly better, but it did prompt me to take action.

I found a counselor and I strongly suggested to John that we go together, at least for a couple of sessions. He didn't believe in counseling, but he went because he saw how much it meant to me. I kept going long after he stopped.

I realized through counseling that John was not completely responsible for my happiness, and I wasn't completely responsible for his. We made adjustments and our church life was a huge piece of that. I had attended a women's retreat called "Christ Renews His Parish," and the men had their own version. One of my non-negotiables was that John had to attend the men's version. I would keep the kids all weekend by myself, but John had to go. He did and he was changed by it. I still have his workbook from that event so many years ago.

We were in Chicago for six long years. For the first three years we were there, my prayer to God every day was "Please, please, please take us back to Dallas. Please, God, take us back to Dallas." Dallas, Texas and I have always been best friends. It has always been my happy place, and since I was so unhappy, I figured why not go to my happy place?

After three years, I stopped praying that prayer. I realized God was going to do what He was going to do, which might not be what Rachel wanted Him to do. I'm not proud of that, because I knew what I wanted, and I thought my plan would be best for me. I had gotten on with my life, made friends, rebuilt my business, and we were involved in church. The boys were doing well, and John and I had overcome the speed bump, and we were okay.

One day, John walked in from work and said, "Guess what? I got a call today and we are going back to Dallas." I said, "Don't mess with me. Do not mess with me about that, because I have put that out of my mind and realized that's not happening." He responded, "No, it's happening." I looked at him, somewhat in shock, and asked, "Are you serious?" He said, with a big grin, "Yes, I'm serious."

When I think of our time in Chicago, I think of the blessings. Reuniting with Pastor Greg and his wife, IdaLynn, was a blessing. Meeting Denise was a blessing. If I had not had those blessings in my life during that time, I shudder to think of what would have happened because I went in and out of depression. Even as I think about it now, I am overcome with emotion about how good our God is. He does hear us. He knows the desires of our hearts. He hears our cries, our pleading, and our begging. Not to say we are always going to get what we want when we want it. Not at all. But in that moment, I was reminded once again about the goodness of God.

Adding to the Family

The arrival of John William Edward Schneider III (aka J3) on February 27, 1997, rocked our world. He was a great baby, a small one at 6 lbs. 7 oz, with a good disposition. A bonus was that my migraines subsided after childbirth. Trixi, our Airedale, was especially excited to welcome him home. My parents had been with us for a while, and they stayed until the end of April. Since they lived in Australia, their visits, though not frequent, tended to be longer than most.

John was the first grandchild on both sides, so he was given extra attention and a lot of responsibility. What? He was to be the bridge between family members who couldn't seem to get along. Here's the story.

John's parents divorced after 26 years of marriage. It was all relatively new when I first met Elaine. Ronald transferred to SMU and moved from California to Dallas to support his mom. John had just accepted a position with an accounting firm in Houston, so he stayed there. John's sister, Cheryl, stayed in California to go to school. John Sr. lived in California with his second wife, Trish.

Elaine met her second husband, Van, who was like the calm in the sea of chaos in which the rest of the family swam. Van was so easy to be around and was curious about everything. He enjoyed reading and contributed to a book about refurbished race cars called *Deuce* because he had restored one when he was younger. He loved the History Channel and was always tinkering with something or working outside. He especially loved taking pictures and the boys were two of his favorite subjects. He would create captions and put them in an album. This was long before Shutterfly. He also enjoyed writing and telling stories. *Bingo, The Horse, and His Adventures* kept the boys entertained for hours.

When it was time to host their annual party at Casa Grande, watch out. Van would spend weeks preparing for that weekend. He hung lights, rearranged furniture, set up an outdoor bar, created misting stations, outdoor TVs, pink parrots, and lots of tables for eating, drinking, playing cards, and Mexican train games. The population of Casa Grande swelled to 50 with air mattresses, rollaway beds, campers, and RVs. I was lucky enough to attend one just by accident, and it lived up to its reputation.

Seniors Gone Wild just about sums it up. One night was about all I could manage. What I did love was that everyone had such a *young-at-heart* attitude, although their bodies might not be in sync with their minds. Recovery time needed to be extended if someone overindulged. The proof is in the pictures and, I may be old-fashioned, or maybe it's the way I was raised, but partying with my or John's parents wasn't anything I wanted or needed to do. Sometimes it's better to hear about things rather than participate in them.

Regardless, Van was well-loved and well-liked. All the men wanted to look like him, with his movie star good looks, and all the women wanted to be Elaine. However, they only had eyes for each other, and anyone who was around them for any length of time knew and felt that. He and Elaine were a package deal, and it was seldom to see one without the other.

We spent more time with John's family, just because of geography, and we tried to maintain good relationships with all of the in-laws. Things got a lot better after Elaine met Van, and John Sr. married Jan.

I remember J3's baptism. Both John Sr. & Jan and Elaine & Van stayed at our house. Ronald chose a hotel, saying that it was all a bit much. I asked John how he felt seeing his mom and dad in their bathrobes, having coffee together in our kitchen. I'm not sure he gave it much thought, but it certainly caused me to think. Remember, I had seen and heard how they talked about and with each other, so I was a bit gun-shy, to say the least. Forty-eight hours would be the extent of a visit. After that, the bickering would start, and it would not be pretty.

Since both John Sr. and Elaine had homes in Palm Desert, we would celebrate Thanksgiving or Christmas with everyone. That's a bit non-traditional, but for the most part, it worked out well.

Four years later, in 2001, we had another son, Jake, who was a gift from God and another reason for me to want to spend more time at home with John, J3, and our new baby.

Losing Ronald

By this time, word of Ronald's condition had gotten out in Dallas, and he was determined to leave. He parted ways with Darren, yet they remained friends. He sold his home in Dallas and gave away his golden retrievers. Both Elaine and Ronald relocated to the Los Angeles area to rebuild their real estate careers. They worked together buying, rehabbing, and selling homes and doing well. My personal favorite was one he never saw but would have loved. Casa Grande is an adorable triplex in Palm Desert situated around a pool, its own oasis in the desert, with easy access to El Paseo, and a wonderful view of the mountains and the fireworks in July. It remains one of my all-time favorite places on earth.

We lived in Naperville for six years, then we headed back to Dallas. I promptly donated all snow boots, parkas, and gloves. We wouldn't need them anymore.

Around this same time, Ronald's condition had morphed into full-blown AIDS. He was able to continue his experimental treatments, but his body was weakening. He took great care of himself and kept a positive attitude. Only his mother, Elaine, knows the full extent of the toll it took on him.

Ronald's sister, Cheryl, decided to take an activist role and cajoled her brother into fundraising appearances to support her two AIDS bike rides. I don't know how Ronald felt about this, but he complied with her requests. John and I were busy raising the boys, so we didn't know how bad he was getting. We found out when Ronald came to visit us in Dallas. He was excited to visit us in the house and be with the boys, but while he was with us, he developed pneumonia. I remember helping him dress as John and I were preparing to take him to the hospital. He was in Lewisville

Hospital for almost two weeks. Both Elaine and John Sr. flew to Dallas to be with him.

Ronald was fading. His body just couldn't fight the double pneumonia that had developed in his chest. Several times we thought he was gone, yet, in the end, he managed to bounce back once again, get cleared by the doctor for release, and within a week of discharge, he was on his way home to Los Angeles. The doctor was surprised at Ronald's stamina and determination to get home. He made his flight reservation, and I helped him get ready for the trip. We got a wheelchair at the airport, I bought him several magazines and snacks, wheeled him down the jetway to board the plane early, kissed him on the forehead, and he gallantly waved me off. This was on a Thursday and the last time I would see him.

The following Saturday night, Elaine called and asked for my squash casserole recipe; Ronald had requested it for dinner. He was staying with her and Van in Long Beach.

She went to wake him the next morning and he was gone. Sometime during the night, so quietly, so silently, so not like Ronald, yet so like Ronald, he slipped away. I didn't ask Van and Elaine what it was like to experience this. I didn't want to upset them, but I wondered how Elaine would answer.

Then, years later, through a conversation, she answered my unspoken question. She shared how they had a lovely dinner that evening and then everybody went to bed. It was an evening not very different from all the others. Elaine said that around four o'clock the next morning, she woke and felt a different presence in the house; an angelic presence. She didn't see anything, yet she sensed a different energy and didn't know why.

When Ronald didn't come for coffee, she checked in on him and found he was gone. She was peaceful, of course, yet so very sad. There wasn't panic or her running through the house, wailing. She had been prepared by what she felt earlier that morning, even though she didn't know what it was about.

Sometimes we get a sense of things, and we don't know why. Yet, we later find out why it happened or why it was good that we honored that sense. Oftentimes, it's the Holy Spirit speaking to us and we aren't even aware of it.

If there's anything I can encourage us to take from this part of the story it is that we need to trust ourselves; to trust in this gift we've been given and recognize that we are a spiritual being living in a human body. The Holy Spirit indwells us and speaks to us, and we need to know, receive, and believe that. It's like Elaine had a peace that passed her ability to understand it, as declared in Philippians 4:7.

> We need to trust ourselves; to trust in this gift we've been given and recognize that we are a spiritual being living in a human body.

After Ronald's death, John and I debated whether to fly to California for the viewing. I wasn't planning on going because I had too much to do, and I was taking care of the boys. Did I mention that I was asked to put together Ronald's memorial service?

How do you put together a memorial service for someone who doesn't have a home church or a pastor? Since John and I were the only ones attending church at that time, we were the likely choice to coordinate and pay for the service. I had hoped that since Ronald was so particular about everything, he would have left instructions on what he wanted. Yet, none were to be found. Except for that one time he joked about having his ashes spread up and down Rodeo Drive or in Highland Park Village in Dallas, with special emphasis at the Cole Haan and Polo stores.

I was flying blind. I thought, well, let's plan a memorial for a gay man who died of AIDS in a Lutheran church he never visited with a pastor who only met him once. That sounded easy enough.

I did pick one spiritual song I knew he would have loved because it was recorded by one of his favorites, Barbra Streisand. It was the hymn, "Standing on Holy Ground."

God knew my heart was in the right place, yet my execution may have left a bit to be desired. I worked through the details while John traveled to California to see his brother, say goodbye, and support his parents. John was scared, unsure, and sad. My heart hurt for him, yet I had no other words than "I'm sorry."

I have learned through the years that sometimes there are just no words. Sometimes there's nothing that can be said, except to share the silence, allow the hurt to be felt, sit with someone in their sorrow, and just be, which can be the hardest thing to do, and something our culture does not embrace or appreciate. Until it's them.

Ronald died a few days short of his 40th birthday. Elaine lost her son. John and Cheryl lost their brother. He lost out on being Uncle Ronnie, something he was so excited about. Our boys meant so much to him, and we know he would have spoiled them rotten.

The service went well, and we had a gathering afterward, which was okay, but a little crowded. We had a tent in the backyard, and we had to cope with the Texas heat in mid-August.

John and I planted flowers the night before in the dark to make things look tip-top. We called it "surprise" gardening because we figured it would be a surprise to see what it looked like in the light of day. Looking back, Ronald would have changed everything, I'm sure of that, but he knew I was going to give it my best, so he granted me some grace.

There were photos, albums, tears, smiles, hugs, and stories.

Through it all, I knew I would probably never see most of the guests again. That's what is said about weddings and funerals, right? I wondered how most of them would remember Ronald and how long they would remember him. I wondered how Elaine would manage. Knowing she had Van made it a little easier, but not much. I thought about how Ronald had lived with such zeal, a carpe diem, and seize the day mentality. I wondered if he had always been like that or if it had manifested with his diagnosis.

> I refuse to believe that God makes people sick.

I believed he was in heaven. I wondered what he thought of it. I knew Ronald believed in God, Jesus, and the Holy Spirit. He knew how I felt about his lifestyle, yet he knew I loved him, and Jesus loved him even more. At one point, I might have believed that gay people deserved AIDS, but I didn't believe that anymore. Ronald helped me see that gay people are people, not some distant aliens needing harsh judgment.

What I did believe, and still do, is that all sin has consequences. Our lives are a result of the choices we make. Sometimes we choose wisely, and sometimes we don't. I hated that the choice Ronald made resulted in this. But there was nothing I could do except pray for and support him the best I knew.

I remember talking with a prayer warrior, telling them about Ronald, and asking them to pray. They said, "No", he brought this on himself through his lifestyle. I was shell-shocked; stunned. How could anyone refuse to pray for someone who was sick? I asked, "What do you think Jesus would do?" Their response was, "Well, it's already been done." As for me, I refuse to believe that God makes people sick. I do believe that he allows us to be tested. Job is a testimony to that. God allowed the devil to do anything except kill Job to test his faith. And Job lost everything. His kids, home, land, herds, and health. Yet he still would not turn on his God.

Maybe Ronald's illness and death were a test for the rest of us. Maybe it was meant to be a wake-up call. It turned out to be a life-changing event that grew my compassion quotient and my ability to look past the sin and see the sinner, which we all are. He made homosexuality real to me, and the awful disease associated with it took away my dear brother-in-law too soon.

Relocating Again | Look out Winter

And then, it was time to move again. It seemed that as soon as I got home from donating all the cold weather gear, John called to tell me about an offer to run a company in Minneapolis. The offer was too good to pass up. It was October 2004, and we were moving again. It's all good, right?

While this was great for John, I was concerned about how I would manage a relocation, my family, and my Partylite business. Of course, we weren't supposed to let anything interfere with our business, yet the reason we chose this direct sales career was for flexibility and freedom.

Yet my days of flexibility and freedom were about to come to a screeching halt!

CHAPTER

3

THE BEGINNING
OF THE END

Minneapolis

The male members of our family adjusted well to the Minnesota move. J3 was in second grade and Jake was in preschool. John was busy working. There I was, trying to find my place... Again. I had built a career in direct sales and most of my team was still in Dallas. I was told that in this virtual world, my relocation would be seamless. I was assured that my team would never even know I was gone. Really?

I was thrilled to have Paula with us. She lived in our basement for a while until she found a beautiful condo to buy. She helped me get things settled in the house and helped with the boys. She was amazing. Paula could be a disciplinarian, a comic, a magician, and she could make a healthy meal and do it all with a beautiful smile on her face. She had a great sense of humor and a razor-sharp wit, which is probably one of the reasons we got along so well. John just ping-ponged between the two of us. She was part of our family. And she juggled all this while working all day at W.D. Larson Companies with John.

I managed to hold it together for a few years before it became apparent that the demands of being a corporate wife with small children tipped the scales. After much soul-searching and talking with God, I parted ways with Partylite. John was thrilled. I didn't need to work, according to him, because he was making good money. There were no worries. Right?

Well, perhaps for a while. Settling into the new northern tundra proved to be a bit more challenging. The Southern hospitality I had grown up with wasn't as evident in the Twin Cities. I couldn't see how the "Minnesota nice" had an element of reality to it. People would wave and smile, but heaven forbid they would invite you in. I had a woman even tell me she had enough friends and didn't need or want anymore. But it's all good... Right?

Nevertheless, we managed to forge ahead, make a few friends, and adapt to our new home. I set up my home office in the three seasons room. When winter hit, because there was no heat in that room, it got cold, but I worked there year-round. I just put on more clothes and plugged in a few more space heaters. It was fine. It had a lot of light, all my books, all my papers, and my desk, which was custom-made to give me plenty of room for all my accoutrement.

Our search for a church home started and stopped, then started again and stopped. Finding the right church has always been one of the most challenging parts of relocation. Right up there with a new doctor and hair stylist. When we didn't have kids, I'll admit, we may have let it slide a bit, but once we became parents, those familial habits kicked in and both of us wanted our boys to be "brought up in the church" just like we were. However, there is a huge difference between "growing up in the church" and having a real relationship with Jesus…right? At least I have found that to be the case for me.

Our search in Minnesota was more of the same, and since we had baptized the boys Lutheran with Pastor Greg in Chicago, we thought it best to start with that denomination. Who knew there were factions within the denomination? It's so conflicted and confusing. I'm glad there won't be any denominations in heaven.

> There is a huge difference between "growing up in the church" and having a real relationship with Jesus…right?

So, after lots of looking, learning, and listening, we landed at Mt. Calvary Lutheran, a mid-size church with both traditional and contemporary services, a Saturday night service, and a curriculum for kids that any parent could desire. What made it even better was that many of the boys' friends attended the church as well, so it became a natural extension of our community.

John was relishing his responsibilities in his new role and working non-stop. After a few summer seasons, he treated himself to his dream—a boat. He asked me to go boat shopping with him. I said, "Honey, I know absolutely nothing about boats. I don't know the difference between a motorboat, a rowboat, and a tugboat. Just make sure you get one with a bathroom and some air conditioning." Which is exactly what he did. It was the biggest boat I had ever seen. The boys were ecstatic and John, a man of simple pleasures, was thrilled. I was overwhelmed yet again. It's all good, right?

I learned that Minnesota is all about the lake—fresh or frozen, fishing on open water or ice, the lake is where it's at. I hadn't grown up with a boat and had no idea how much work they could be. Storing, prepping, supplying, cleaning, entertaining, fueling, docking—the list of chores seemed endless. A few friends took pity on me and shared their boat management systems, which saved so much time in the years that came. Eventually, I did learn to enjoy our time on the lake.

John shared his love of water with our sons—J3 learned to drive and dock the boat like a pro. The boys and Dad bonded tightly on the "The Three J's" and, for that, I will always be grateful.

The Diagnosis

The year was 2008 and John's symptoms showed themselves almost in a stealth-like manner. He had always been an athlete and was inclined to brush off minor strains and unusual aches. He thought it was a simple pull of the hamstring. Perhaps one foot on the dock, the other in the boat had caused an unexpected pull and other annoying symptoms. However, over a period of time, these symptoms were not going away, and they were not getting any better.

In secret, John started to see a neurologist and he kept seeing that neurologist for more than a year. As the strength in his left side declined, he knew it wasn't a pulled hamstring like he had originally thought. After consulting a colleague, John's doctor sent him home with a diagnosis. It was on a Friday and the doctor knew John was scheduled for his executive physical at the Mayo Clinic the following Monday. The doctor thought John should take his chart with him and have the physicians at the Mayo Clinic offer their expertise. So, John came home with all that information in the file.

My sister, Nicole, and I are only 15 months apart. We had not been close since the beginning of her marriage—some four years earlier. It wasn't anything ugly, it was just a distance that turned into a rift that then turned into a gulf. It happened that, at the same time as John's doctor appointment, Nicole had made plans to visit Minneapolis—pretty unusual for her since she lived in Hawaii. Her husband's family lives in Cleveland, so she decided to pay a quick visit on her way back home. John realized how much the weekend with my sister could mean. He completely supported giving us whatever "girl time" we needed. Little did I know what John was already going through.

That night John stayed late at the office. Nicole and I had plans to have a nice dinner out and get caught up while he stayed home and watched the boys. He arrived home late, and I was upset because it seemed like he was always about work. There is always another fire to put out, some other crisis to counter.

He walked in looking frazzled, but I wasn't paying that much attention. Nicole and I left him with the boys and headed out to a lovely dinner. We reconnected over that weekend, spending time with John and the boys, playing games, and relaxing. There was a genuine feeling of coming together again. It was heartfelt and a divine restoration for us.

Knowing what information the folder contained, John kept it to himself because he didn't want to interfere with my weekend plans. That is who John was. This was the character of my husband and how truly caring he was. Restoring our sister relationship was just one of the gifts he gave us.

This is America—where anything is possible!

The weekend ended, my sister left, and John headed to the Mayo Clinic in Rochester, Minnesota, by himself with files in hand. He was planning to stay overnight in Rochester, so I was surprised when he called me and said he was coming home. He told me the doctors wanted me to be there for some of the tests the next day. I thought it was an odd request and suggested that he stay and rest awhile. I would drive down and meet him the next morning. He insisted that he wanted to come home so we could drive together the next day.

When I hung up the phone, I didn't think too much about it. The boys were asleep, and I was tucked in and reading a book when John came home. He looked frightened and was as white as a ghost. He came over to my side of the bed, sat down and said, "They think I have this disease, ALS. And I'm going to die." He couldn't catch his breath. I said, "Wait a minute, slow down. What are you talking about?" He said, "They think I have this disease, ALS, Lou Gehrig's disease. I'm going to die."

I looked at him and asked, "What is ALS? Die? It can't be THAT bad." I mean, let's not get overdramatic. Yet something resonated deep within my soul since John was not a man given to drama or overstating the case. He had always been calm, cool, and collected—which had served him well during his years of climbing the corporate ladder. So, when he told me the doctors wanted me to be there with him the next day, I didn't hesitate.

I had no idea what was before us.

We'll go show those doctors, I thought. They can't be right about this and even if they are, there has got to be something we can do about it. After all, this is America—where anything is possible! Where we set the standard for so many things, especially medical technology and medical miracles. And better yet, we have God on our side and with Him all things are possible, right?

I comforted John as best I could and encouraged him to get some sleep, noting that we would talk more about this the next day. Who knew we would spend the next three years talking about nothing else.

The Mayo Clinic

The drive was uneventful. John was on the phone most of the time since he had been given the tough task of cutting expenses quickly—which was code for letting a few people go and cutting the pay for those who remained. His assistant and my good friend, Paula, had already started looking for a part-time job to supplement the cut in her full-time income. This process had taken a toll on John, and it didn't help that it was so close to Thanksgiving. Everyone in the office knew he was going in for his executive physical appointment.

The main complex is about a two-hour drive from where we lived. A city within a city, the Mayo Clinic is known worldwide for being the "mothership of medicine." Celebrities, world leaders, and politicians come from all over the world to be treated at the Mayo Clinic in Rochester, Minnesota. The huge campus consists of the Mayo and the Gonda building, which houses the ALS Clinic. The rest of the city is made up of a host of specialty medical and therapeutic services and supplies, hotels, restaurants, short-term rentals, literally everything and anything you can think of that would be needed in the health and wellbeing arena. The entire town was designed with ease of treatment and accessibility in mind.

The Gonda building was named after Mr. Gonda, a benefactor of many medical institutions, museums, and charities. He donated to the learning center at the Holocaust Museum in Washington, and he is a native Hungarian who survived the Holocaust. He immigrated to Venezuela where he started a business leasing airplanes. He then moved his family and business to Los Angeles.

The campus is huge. It has a breast diagnostic center, children's center, dental specialties, gastroenterology, hepatology, ear, nose and throat, executive health program, bing, bing, bing, that's where John started. Infectious diseases, general internal medicine, sleep medicine, and women's health. Last but not least, it has a cafeteria, pharmacy, retail shops, and supplies. (By the way, I have done some of my best shopping at airports and hospitals.) It is enormous. They have beautiful accommodations for people to stay for days, weeks, or months while they get their treatment.

We found our way to meet with Dr. Stephanie Faubion who seemed as surprised as we were to be heading to neurology for some additional tests. After all, how many times did a 47-year-old business executive walk into her office only to be diagnosed with a terminal illness with a life expectancy of two to five years? I daresay we were the first.

She was as surprised as we were two days later when the tests were completed, and the diagnosis was confirmed. They were checking for twitching, they were checking for muscle mass, strength, and all that stuff. We got to the car; I think it was six o'clock at night. He looked at me and he said, "I have a headache." I looked at him and said, "I have a heartache." We were both just devastated.

So, let me pause here and give a brief explanation of ALS, Amyotrophic Lateral Sclerosis. The short answer is that it's a nervous system disease that affects nerve cells in the brain and spinal cord, causing loss of muscle control.

For the longest time, I didn't want to speak the name because I didn't want to give it any kind of power. Now that I've walked through it with John, I have a better understanding and will break it down a little for the reader. Amyotrophic is derived from the Greek word meaning no muscle nourishment, so this refers to the atrophy of the muscles, which is caused by the lack of neural input. Lateral refers to the areas of the spinal cord where the motor neurons are located. Sclerosis is the hot scarring or hardening that happens as the motor neurons degenerate.

Here's how it affects the body. The motor neurons, which are the cells that transmit the signals from the brain to the muscles and enable voluntary movements, are where the disease targets, causing them to die. As neurons die, communication between both the brain and the muscle is disrupted, causing progressive muscle weakness and paralysis. It can also create frontotemporal dementia. Because the diaphragm is a muscle, it stops working, which is eventually what causes death. The patient suffocates.

About 5,500 people each year are diagnosed in the United States with ALS. An estimated 13-40% of patients get feeding tubes, and less than 15% receive a tracheostomy. Our medical system is still managing a disease that has no known cause or cure.

ALS is Lou Gehrig's disease, named after the well-known baseball player. The disease had presented itself before in others, but because of his celebrity, he got more attention. Doctors studied his symptoms and were able to figure out what was going on. Lou Gehrig was quite the baseball player. He played for the New York Yankees and was a celebrated athlete with the nickname "The Iron Horse" because of his durability and his consecutive game streak of 2,130 games.

After being diagnosed with ALS, he had to leave the world of baseball. At his last game, he shared these words, "I consider myself to be one of the luckiest men alive." He was diagnosed at the age of 35 in 1939; he died in 1941 which meant he fell in the middle of the two to five-year timeline. At that time, ALS didn't have a lot of

"Go home, have a glass of wine, hold on to each other, and try to let this go for a while."

recognition; because of Lou Gehrig and his fame, the disease was attributed to him. Lou Gehrig's disease remains a very common term. It serves as a tribute to his courage and his resilience in the face of the illness. When we look back at his life, it speaks well to the moniker.

As I began to grasp the brutality of this disease, I knew that getting the best in every aspect of treatment was important. The psychological, emotional, mental, and spiritual components had to be addressed. My biggest concern with the visits to the Mayo Clinic, the ALS clinic housed there, and any ALS clinic across the country, was how they lacked the spiritual component. With a diagnosis like this, there should be some discussion about faith and support, or at least acknowledgment of the role faith plays in a treatment or healing process.

What did we get from Dr. Faubion? "Go home, have a glass of wine, hold on to each other, and try to let this go for a while."

Oh, if it had only been that easy.

4

NEVER A GOOD WAY TO SHARE BAD NEWS

Decisions

After I heard John's news, there was shock followed by this all-encompassing numbness that took over. To find answers, I overwhelmed myself with too much information. I went to the Minneapolis ALS headquarters and asked, "What do we do? What have you got? What kind of resources? Where do I go? How can you help?" They were nice, even though I didn't find what I was looking for. I just wanted somebody to give me the options, tell me what to investigate, or connect us with someone. Perhaps they were overwhelmed too. I don't know how they do what they do. I left with a lot of pamphlets, brochures, information about meetings, a set of books, and a guidebook.

Then I went to the internet to check out different kinds of

alternative treatments. This was also overwhelming, but it's where I learned more about stem cell treatments. I had heard about celebrities who went to Germany for these treatments, which were seen as experimental in our country. John and I discussed it a bit. We didn't think about it a whole lot because at that time he wasn't symptomatic. This was a discussion for another time and another phase of the disease.

We did make decisions about who to tell, when to tell, and how to tell people the news. But first, we wanted to go to the throne of God. Joyce Meyer says, "Go to the throne before you go to the phone." That's the way John and I have lived, both individually and as a couple. We were walking through this with Jesus. John, Jesus, and me.

We didn't live near our family, and we had moved around so much. My parents and brothers were in Australia and had been for years. My sister was in Hawaii. We communicated through Skype, but we didn't keep up with day-to-day life. We talked about the big things.

John's parents were divorced and lived on the West Coast with new spouses. We couldn't just drive over. So, John and I learned how to navigate with just one another. It had always been that way and through the years, it became even more natural. When anything happened, we figured it out for ourselves.

There were several reasons we needed to figure things out on our own. First, we knew from our family dynamics that we needed to be on the same page. Second, both of us were the eldest children. There are character traits of the firstborn, one of which is responsibility. As our siblings came along, we had a protective nature about them. We didn't mean to be competitive or set a high standard, but we were, and we did. And we were the ones the parents were careful with, because everything about being parents of the firstborn was new for them, too.

John and I took our responsibility as firstborn children seriously. It was an innate quality we had. It was our job to figure things out. Now, this situation left us without words, speech, or comprehension, and we didn't know where to go to get this figured out. It's one thing to get a somewhat common diagnosis. I don't say that with ease, and I don't mean it lightly. Cancer is common. Diabetes is common. Hypertension is common. Heart issues are common. But ALS isn't common. (Thank God for that!) There's nothing about it that's normal. And there's nothing about that uncommon quality that lessens the magnitude of the moment. It's big.

ALS is not a diagnosis any doctor wants to give. And it's not a diagnosis any person wants to get. Figuring out what to do with this information took a while. It was early November 2008, a dark, dreary, and desolate day in Minnesota. The beginning of what was supposed to be the most wonderful time of the year, and yet the most depressing if you're not into snow, cold, ice, blizzards, and wind. And I wasn't. I just wasn't.

For me, winter in Minnesota was the time to get out. I always looked forward to our trips to see Elaine in Palm Desert. We had been going there since J3 was a baby and I loved everything about it. John and Cheryl never enjoyed the desert, but Ronald and I loved it. It's like an older version of Dallas with lots of shopping, pools, and people-watching. The sun. Sherman's Deli, a great Jewish delicatessen. The beauty of the mountains. The social atmosphere. Stein Mart. It was always such a fun time. And did I mention how much fun Ronald was shopping with? I never set foot in SAKS unless I was with him. He picked out a marvelous red suit, jacket with gold buttons, and skirt above the knee, and he insisted I wear it with pumps and lots of pearls, a la Coco Chanel. The suit is long gone, yet I can remember that outing and every time I wore that suit, I not only looked great; I also felt great.

But this particular year, I dreaded the trip.

I shared the news over the phone with Nicole and shared how John had kept his diagnosis under wraps so we could have our sister's weekend. She burst into tears. She couldn't believe he had done that for us. With her background, she became a resource as John progressed through his illness. She provided insights into nutrition, feeding tubes, and home and hospice care. While we live different lifestyles, she was there for me.

With my parents and my two brothers living in Australia, we realized that we could share this information with them and not worry about it going anywhere else. And we knew, I knew, that I desperately needed their prayers, their support. I needed them to share with their prayer partners and church family about John's illness. We needed prayers for healing and strength.

We decided to place the call from my office. Australia is on the other side of the world, and their time frame is different, so we made the call at night. It was around 8 p.m. our time and mid-morning for them. When John got on the call, they knew right away that something was up because he was never on the call. Also, I had requested that all of them be together.

We didn't waste any time getting to the point. John and I both have always been straightforward in relaying information and delivering the news of his diagnosis was no different. I still can't pronounce the scientific word, *amyotrophic lateral sclerosis*. It's ALS or Lou Gehrig's disease. And usually, people can get it from that.

My parents were not sure they had heard of it. I think my brother James had. After we knew they understood what we were talking about, we then proceeded to give them more information.

We gave as much information as we could, which was his body was going to self-paralyze and that he had between two and five years to live. We didn't get overly dramatic about it. I didn't hear anything from my mother; she was off-camera just a little. I asked, "Mom, are you okay?" James said, "She's emoting right now." He has such a way with words. I had to smile. Other than that, I can't say there was a lot of external emotion emitted.

We were emotional, but I've never been given over to bouts of tears or anger. I don't throw things. I don't scream. I don't yell. I don't stomp around and slam doors. I've never been prone to fits of crying either. So, the entire call was fairly matter-of-fact in relaying the information to my mother, father, and two brothers. While the message was devastating, the way it was delivered was standard operating procedure for me.

My mom and dad were supportive and said something like this. "When you call, we will be there, but we will wait for you to call. We understand you and John have your own life. You have been married for a long time, and we haven't been involved to a certain degree. But when you're ready for us to come, we will be there. And when we come, we are going to stay there and see this through." I heard what they were saying, and I believed them. But for now, I wasn't ready. I could do this. I wasn't the first person to have to walk through this and, with God's strength, we would make it through.

Who to Share With and When to Share

We didn't want our boys to know yet. John still looked healthy and there wasn't anything about his physique that had changed. Maybe if someone knew and looked, they would notice his left foot wasn't as mobile as the right one, but it wasn't keeping him from doing anything. He was the only one truly aware of it. And our boys were so young. We just knew holding the news from them was the right thing to do. The decision was made almost immediately; we didn't agonize over it. We were both sure. We knew the right time would present itself, and we were going to wait until John became more symptomatic.

Sharing the information with John's parents would be a new ballgame and we weren't ready to deal with them, quite honestly. We decided to spend the holiday in the warm desert with John's family and tell them while we were there. We had celebrated Christmas in the snow in Minnesota for a lot of years. We made the best reindeer food, enjoyed concerts, and marveled at the twinkling lights. We did all the things people do to incorporate the frozen tundra into their lives. But I preferred the sunshine and warmth. Considering what was going on, this seemed like a good year to get away and would give us a better place to share our news. Elaine and Van had a home in the desert and so did John Sr. and Jan. John Sr. and Jan's primary residence was in San Jose. It sounds odd and, indeed, it was highly unusual that all of us would see each other and spend a fair amount of time together during the holidays. But that's what we did.

Tickets were booked. The boys and I would arrive two days ahead of John, which wasn't unusual. He always had work, and I was excited to bask in the sunshine of the desert. But before Christmas rolled around, we received more devastating news to share.

Decimated

In mid-December, John was let go from his position. The timing was two weeks after his diagnosis and two weeks before Christmas. It was a strange coincidence since no one at his company knew about his illness. John had been agonizing for two weeks about letting people go and cutting salaries. It was all happening before, during, and after Thanksgiving, with some layoffs taking place before Christmas.

John was the hatchet man, but what he didn't know was that soon he was going to be chopped up as well. He was equally devastated, blindsided, and shocked when he was let go, his assistant, and my best friend Paula, was let go, and the chief financial officer that he had hired was let go. All three in one day. I was devastated for him. The ALS diagnosis was like getting run over by a truck. Losing his job was like having the truck back up and run over us again. It was a miracle we were still standing or breathing.

This was a strange situation to be in since John had never been let go of any job, ever. Let's just call it what it was. Fired: it was brutal. For John, providing for his family was everything. And in our culture, our identity is wrapped up in our job title and what we do. It was everything he wanted in his professional career. He was running a company with 650 employees, and six or seven different locations, and he was the boss. He had been named by the owner of the company to run the business; he was also the only person who could let him go. For John, it was devastating, probably even more so than the news about the disease, at least for a while.

This was the beginning of a very traumatic time in our lives. Shortly after, Paula was diagnosed with cervical cancer and our relationship began to unravel. It wasn't anyone's fault. She chose to deal with her cancer in her way, and I had to step back and respect her wishes. There's a fine line when someone is going through difficulties, whether it's a health challenge, a job challenge, or a relationship challenge. All I could do was pray and support her in whatever way I could until it became clear that my support wasn't welcomed or needed.

The Word of the Day: Numb

I was numb for months. I wasn't sure about the job situation – maybe John didn't need to work anyway. We would be okay, or would we? Should we sell the house, go somewhere, live quietly, scale things back?

In truth, we had no game plan for the loss of his job. Interestingly enough, John chose to share the information about the job loss with his parents before we got there for the holiday. They were prepared that it might be a different kind of Christmas with John in transition and focused on finding another job. They just didn't know how different it was going to be. The job was just part of the story; the other information was the real zinger.

John and I were completely united that we would not wreck the holiday any more than we had already. I don't know why I'm taking responsibility, or John either. It wasn't our fault at all. I guess that's what firstborns do. I constantly worried about keeping our lives as normal as possible when the world was crashing around us. This was no time for my resilience muscle to lose its strength. Things were just getting started.

Reflections: Relationship Challenges

Some relationships are meant to last a lifetime, while others are only with us for a season. As painful as it is, we have to listen when God whispers that a chapter is closing. Not every friendship can be revived once it fades, and sometimes, no matter how much we wish it could, the bond just doesn't hold.

When Paula and I drifted apart, I felt the weight of her absence in every part of my life. I missed her laughter, the way we could talk for hours, and the comfort of knowing she was always there. She was woven into so many of my memories and letting go wasn't easy. But even in the ache of separation, gratitude remained. She had been a beautiful part of my journey, a gift from God for that season. And while friendships may change, the love and lessons they leave behind never truly fade.

When my relationship with Paula began to unravel, I had to make one of the hardest choices - to honor her wishes and step back. It broke my heart. Our lives had been woven together for so long, through every joy and every storm. She wasn't just a friend. She was family. But not all relationships are meant to last forever. Some are gifts for a season, shaping us, teaching us, and then painfully slipping away.

I've learned to trust that gentle nudge from the Holy Spirit, the quiet whisper that tells us when to hold on and when to let go. Sometimes, He stirs our hearts to reconnect, guiding us back to someone in His perfect timing. Other times, no matter how much we long to bridge the distance, He gently but firmly closes the door. Not out of cruelty, but out of love, because He sees what we cannot. And in those moments, as much as it hurts, I've found peace in surrendering to His will, believing that every goodbye is making room for something greater ahead.

Reflections: Jesus, Our Rock, Foundation, and Strong Tower

During that season of uncertainty, one thing never wavered. I knew God was with us. I clung to that truth with everything in me. I believed, I declared, I stood on scripture, convinced that if I prayed hard enough, claimed healing boldly enough, and immersed myself in His word, then surely God would heal John. I surrounded myself with words of power: sermons, books, magazines, Bible studies, and every message from the great voices of the Word of Faith movement. I went to revivals, lifted my hands in worship under the glow of stadium lights, and sat front and center, hungry for every ounce of wisdom I could absorb.

Looking through my journals from that time, I was struck by the intensity of it all. I had forgotten just how deeply I had thrown myself into that world. And while I have no shame in it— no embarrassment—I do recognize now that it was a journey, a migration of sorts, one that reshaped my understanding of faith, prayer, and my relationship with Jesus.

Through it all, I learned a profound truth: what we think we know, and what we've been taught, isn't always the full picture. It is up to us to go deeper, to seek Him beyond what others say, and to recognize that even within Christianity, there are many voices and perspectives. Some are rooted in truth, but some are not. Discernment is essential. We must always approach our faith with both passion and wisdom, holding fast to God's Word as our foundation and allowing the Holy Spirit to be our guide.

As I walked this journey, I realized something profound. The road to knowing Jesus doesn't widen with time; it narrows. The distractions fade, the noise quiets, and my heart becomes fixed on one thing: doing the work to know Him more. That's why we have the Bible—not just as a book of history or poetry, but as a living, breathing lifeline. It became my anchor, my daily bread, and my guide through every storm and every season of growth.

I discovered that spending time with Him wasn't about rigid rules or obligations; it was about relationship. And that relationship deepened through:

- **Reading the Bible** in a way that truly spoke to me, not out of duty but out of hunger.
- **Listening to Scripture** through a Bible app when my eyes or heart were too weary to read.
- **Weaving God's Word into my Daily Life**, making it a rhythm rather than a task.
- **Learning His Promises and Provisions**, understanding that His Word is filled with love, hope, power, and mercy.
- **Discovering His Will for His Children**, knowing that He calls us to freedom and victory, and understanding how He delivers us from the enemy's grip.
- **Strengthening My Spirit**, because the stronger our spirit, the more resilient we become—ready, equipped, and unshaken by life's challenges.

The more I pressed in, the more I realized that knowing Jesus isn't just about reading words on a page. It's about letting those words come alive in me. It's about transformation, about leaning into His truth, about becoming someone who doesn't just know about Him, but someone who truly knows Him. And that, more than anything, has changed everything.

The Holy Spirit is our Comforter, our Guide, our Source of unshakable peace. He is the kind of peace that cannot be found in this world, a peace that surpasses all understanding (Philippians 4:7). Jesus knew we would need Him. He knew that after His crucifixion, when the world turned dark and hope seemed lost, His followers would need a Helper.

After rising from the tomb in a life-altering, earth-shaking moment, Jesus revealed Himself to over 500 people. He stood among them, alive, victorious, and yet, He told His disciples something they didn't expect—He wasn't staying. Imagine their grief, their confusion. They had just begun to grasp the miracle of His resurrection, and now He was leaving... Again? But Jesus didn't leave them empty or abandoned. He gave them a promise: *"I will ask the Father, and He will give you another Comforter, who will never leave you"* (John 14:16). That Comforter was the Holy Spirit, who came in power at Pentecost (Acts 2), filling the disciples with the boldness to carry the gospel across the world, to make disciples, to change history (Matthew 28).

And here's the incredible truth. That same Spirit lives in you. If you believe in Jesus Christ, the power of the Holy Spirit dwells within you. The same Spirit that raised Jesus from the dead, the same Spirit that transformed fearful men into fearless preachers, the same Spirit that continues to move and work today: He is within you.

I won't pretend to understand all the mysteries of the Trinity, of how God, Jesus, and the Holy Spirit work together in perfect unity. But I do know this: it works. And I also know that the Holy Spirit doesn't always get the attention He deserves. So, dear reader, let this be your reminder: His power is real, His presence is here, and He is in you—just as Jesus said.

- Get to know the Holy Spirit.
- Take a moment to read Acts 2:1-21. Let the words sink in. This is where it all began—where the Holy Spirit came like a mighty rushing wind, filling the disciples and changing everything.
- Now, pause. Journal your thoughts. Who is the Holy Spirit to you? How has He moved in your life? How has He comforted you, guided you, or spoken to your heart? If you've never journaled before, I encourage you to try. It doesn't have to be perfect, and you don't have to write every day—but there is something powerful about putting your thoughts on paper and seeing how God is working in your life.

I remember when we lived in our house in Minnesota, the trees stretched high into the sky, it was like living in a treehouse. When the wind would blow—and it did often—I would just sit and listen. Sometimes, it whispered through the trees, and at other times it roared; bending the trees but never breaking them, its presence undeniable. And in those moments, I could feel the Holy Spirit.

To me, the wind is the most tangible, breathtaking representation of the Holy Spirit's power. Invisible, yet mighty. Unseen, yet undeniable. Moving where He wills, filling the world with His presence, reminding us that He is here, always.

SECTION II

FINDING STRENGTH THROUGH THE STORM

"Strengthen your feeble arms and weak knees. Make level paths for your feet, so that the lame may not be disabled, but rather healed."

HEBREWS 12:12-13

CHAPTER

5

ANOTHER DIMENSION TO THE DRAMA

By the time the boys and I got to California, I was wiped out. I didn't look so great. John's family thought it was because of John's employment situation. When John arrived, he didn't look so great either. His family told him things like, "You'll get another job," and "You're going to be fine." I kept thinking how his job was the least of our worries. It just didn't seem important.

Christmas: Kerr-Family Style: The Nativity

As I was growing up, the holidays were celebrated, and the house was decorated but not overdone like we see today. We had a tree with a nativity scene under it; it was simple holiday décor. My mom made it in ceramics class. Because she spent many years in Germany as a Ukrainian refugee of World War II, the nativity kept her focused on the true gift of Christmas and reminded us that the rest of the gifts didn't matter. The gift of Jesus is plenty. He's the greatest gift of all. That's why she placed it under the tree. Maybe it's a European thing or maybe it's a believer thing. I don't know. I'm wondering where other people put their nativity. I haven't seen many under the tree.

I have the nativity my mother painted so many years ago. I'm excited to put it in its place under the Christmas tree. It reminds me of my mom: she's artistic, beautiful, and a gift to us all. When I think of what I learned from her, I'm filled with happiness. She taught me that receiving a lot of gifts wasn't warranted, needed, or necessary. We already have the most wonderful gift of all.

As we grew up and got older, our parents gave us family trips. There were four children, so a trip was a large gift. We were invited to be guests at a lodge in Michigan for several years in a row. My dad did business with the company that owned it. Being from the South, the only skiing I knew was water skiing. I wasn't any good at that, so I knew I wouldn't be any good at snow skiing either. After Michigan, it became cruises, which was a wonderful way to be together but not on top of each other. We were in the same place, same time, but not together 24/7. Cruising was quite the hit. It checked a lot of boxes.

And then I got married. I was the first Kerr child to get married, which changed everything, including the holiday schedule. Marriage introduced a new family with its own culture filled with traditions and a schedule. Nothing stayed the same. And then kids came along, and everything changed again.

I carried the nativity tradition into my marriage with John as a statement that Christmas is not about gifts. It's about the birth of Jesus; the nativity. Because we get a lot during the year, I don't feel a mad rush to put a lot of stuff under the tree. The nativity is all we need. I have always decorated the table beautifully... No matter the holiday or occasion, the table decoration begins a week before, using china, crystal, and cloth napkins. This tradition brings me great joy.

Christmas: Schneider Style

The Schneiders celebrate Christmas with gifts, gifts, and more gifts. I had to get used to it because I was entering a new dimension. Then, as the kids came and the holiday became a joint celebration in the desert, the focus shifted and the gifts would be for the kids, which was fabulous. We still had great dinners, we were in the desert, and being there always made things better.

In 2008, we got through the holiday; we had Christmas. It was one of those holidays that was just difficult. And yet John and I were determined to find joy in the season, which was a struggle. We were also dealing with a situation that was sad, shocking, surprising, disappointing, life-changing, and downright scary. This holiday season was wrecking me because the rug was pulled out from under both of us.

> Watching the holiday unfold was like an out-of-body experience for us.

We planned to take comfort in the routine of how we always celebrated Christmas in the desert. It was a place where we could let things be. We weren't in charge, which was the true gift for that Christmas. John and I could go and take care of one another, which is what we did because the boys were being watched, loved, and spoiled by the Schneider family.

Watching the holiday unfold was like an out-of-body experience for us. Yet we knew it was surreal in that it was normal or at least appeared to be. We were doing our best to maintain the norm all the while knowing it would never be the same.

Telling Elaine, Van, and Cheryl

The day after Christmas, we were at Elaine and Van's house. We asked their friend, Dave, to take the boys out for breakfast. Elaine was sitting on a beautiful, long, gorgeous, exquisite sofa. Van was in the wingback chair. John and I sat with them and told them about John's diagnosis. The moment we said "ALS," Van understood because he had a friend who also had ALS. After Van explained to Elaine that it was the same thing his friend had, she understood.

I didn't cry but John was emotional; his voice broke, and he teared up. I was more concerned about him. We didn't want to share too much because we were still in a state of shock. Hearing the two to five-year life expectancy throws everything else out the window. I was also trying to discern how Elaine was taking the news. Remember, she was getting information that her firstborn son had a terminal disease. She had lost her other son, Ronald, seven years earlier.

Elaine and Van were shocked, numb. But nobody fell apart. We just didn't do that. Van was a Dutchman and good at holding back his emotions. Elaine has a positive outlook about everything, so I wasn't sure she understood quite yet. But we gave them the information just like it had been imparted to us, and then we let it sit for a while. Then, Elaine held John, her oldest son, and he cried on her shoulder. That was difficult.

Soon after, Cheryl arrived. She lived in Los Angeles but was staying with her dad in the desert during the holidays. The boys were still gone. We sat at the circular kitchen table. John sat on one side, I sat on the other, and Cheryl sat between us. Elaine was getting coffee, and Van was standing at the counter. John shared the news with Cheryl and her reaction was pretty standard. She was angry; she knew exactly what ALS was, and we didn't have to explain anything to her. Her job was in sports training, and she was well-educated in things concerning the body, disease, and health. Elaine hugged her daughter and said, "It's going to be fine. It's going to be okay."

Cheryl jumped out of her chair and responded, "This is not going to be fine, Mom. This is not going to be okay." She was almost yelling. And with that, to our surprise, she stormed out, got in her Mercedes, and drove back to Los Angeles. Later she phoned and said, "I can't be with you guys. I need to be by myself. I will catch up with you later." And that was that. She was gone.

Within half an hour, Dave brought the boys back. They played with John in the front yard, roughhousing a bit. That same day, someone delivered a bouquet of the most gorgeous flowers to Elaine. I thought it was a belated Christmas delivery, but it was from Cheryl's partner, Jay. At the time, it struck me as different that he would send a beautiful bouquet to cheer her up after getting such devastating news. Now, it makes sense.

The next day, Cheryl raced back with books about a gentleman who was winning his battle with ALS, *Eric is Winning*. We all read it. Well, John didn't. We were learning about Eric Edney.

Telling John Sr. and Jan

At this point, John and I were exhausted and ready to drop. I don't know how John got through these discussions. The word I kept coming back to was *numb*. I knew God would get us through, but

I didn't know how. I didn't have a clue, and it was past the point of comprehension.

Despite the fact that we were exhausted and numb, we still needed to tell John Sr. and Jan so they would hear it from us the same day as we told the others. We drove to their house and when we arrived, the television was on, and they were watching a ballgame. They served drinks to everyone. John Sr. thought he and my husband were going to work out the whole employment thing. John's dad considered himself somewhat of an expert in finding jobs because he had been in venture capital for a while, meaning he moved from different companies as they were funded to help them grow and prosper. He finished his career in a senior position with Hewlett-Packard. He was going to impart wisdom, perspective, and knowledge to John about his prospects, his search, and of course, they were going to rehash his being expelled from the company as well.

His dad asked, "Do you have any leads for a job?" John waited a minute or so and answered, "I have something I need to tell you." I was waiting for someone to turn down the volume on the television or for John's dad to sit down. But neither of those things happened. So, John said, "I have been diagnosed with ALS."

John Sr. didn't know what to say. I don't think Jan knew what it was either. John gave them more information and his dad asked, "Okay, so how do they treat that?" I was still waiting for the television to be turned off, for the ballgame to end, waiting for somebody to realize life had stopped for a minute and the ballgame wasn't as important as what John was trying to tell them. But that didn't happen. I watched my husband try to explain that there was no cure. Nothing could be done. Still, his dad didn't get it, and John was trying to help him understand. My heart was breaking. Finally, his dad got it, or part of it, and Jan immediately asked if we had enough life insurance.

The ballgame was still going. We were drinking our drinks. We had just dealt devastating news about John's health and lifespan, and she wanted to know if we had enough life insurance. I thought, well, there you have it. That went pretty much the way I thought it would.

Hoping for More

At the time of Ronald's illness and death, I hoped there would be a spiritual wake-up call within the Schneider family. Maybe everyone would get their affairs in order. Maybe they would rely on Jesus a little more. Maybe they would go to church regularly or attend services other than Easter and Christmas.

But no. Here we were with another terminal diagnosis, another bolt of lightning striking another son down, and they were still in the same place. John and I were in a better place spiritually than we had ever been. We attended church and were involved. We had stayed connected with Pastor Greg, who was faithful in praying for us daily.

Everyone in the Schneider family always considered me the "religious one." Here we were in another "only a miracle will do" situation. I don't remember any of them saying, "Okay, let's pray about this, Rachel. Let's talk to Jesus about it right now." That was left up to me and John, but mostly me. I was diligent in praying. I believed John would be healed of ALS, because miracles do still happen. Please know that. I didn't stop believing in John being healed of ALS for a long time. My ability to believe kept me confident, living in the present, and hoping for the future.

CHAPTER

6

FINDING OUR FOOTING

A Change of Lifestyle

Cheryl is a take-charge kind of gal, and she truly believed her way was best. John had grown up with her, so he certainly knew her better. My exposure to her had been limited. So, for a while, I thought she knew best. She does know a lot, and there are subject areas in which she has genuine expertise. She is disciplined and smart when it comes to physical fitness and nutrition.

After reading the book, *Eric is Winning*, the following January, Cheryl swooped in and brought in what she thought our new diet would look like, which was also one of the alternative treatments for dealing with disease. I think the book inspired her to clean up our nutrition, detox our bodies, and see if that might slow ALS down. The food was to be all organic, with no sugar, no carbs, nothing processed, and no white flour. Oh, my goodness.

Fifteen years ago, this was cutting edge, very few people were eating this way. Today this is considered the norm. No big deal. However, it was a big deal to make meals from scratch every day and every night and to pay attention to every bite. John wasn't a fan of eggplant ragu or quinoa, and neither were the boys. It became quite the challenge, but Cheryl was up to it. She continued to do this throughout his illness and got us on this program. John and I both dropped 15 pounds by switching to this clean diet.

When John went back to the Mayo Clinic, he was weighed. They said, "You've lost weight. You don't need to lose any more. How did you do that?" John answered, "Well, I've been eating clean." They responded, "Well, you don't need to lose any more weight." He said, "Oh, okay." They didn't give him any positive reinforcement or encouragement for having lost weight.

When another gal came in, she said, "We haven't met. I'm a nutritionist. When we need to talk about a feeding tube, I'll be the person you see." I was mortified. He could still eat and here we were talking about a feeding tube! Then she told him, "You don't need to lose any more weight, and you don't need to pay attention to your diet.

"There are books out there, *Feed Your Brain,* and there's another book written by a guy we are not even sure has ALS, *Eric is Winning,* she said. Her tone for everything other than what they recommended was completely dismissive. It's as if these books or these people lacked any value whatsoever.

I thought I was going to fall off the chair. I asked, "How do you know that?" She replied, "Well, he's just been alive for too long, and we're not sure he's got the right diagnosis." I looked at her, wondering if she was deliberately trying to extinguish every ounce of hope.

I went home that night and wrote an email to Eric. I'm sure he gets thousands of emails and people contacting him all the time.

I wrote, "I just want you to know that they have heard about you at the Mayo Clinic. They know who you are, they know about your book, and they don't think you have ALS. I was appalled when they told me that today at our clinic visit. I wanted to commend you for what you're doing, for getting the word out, and for successfully fighting this battle like you have all these years."

I didn't expect to get a reply because he's ill and I know his time at the computer is valuable. But he did write back. He said, "It's good to know they have heard about me at the Mayo Clinic. It's sad to know what they think." I thought, how appropriate.

For the reader seeking answers to alternative treatments for illness, I want to devote the next three paragraphs to this topic. Eric Edney is the author, and his wife, Glenna, contributed to the book as well. He wrote a follow-up book, *Surviving Without Your MD*. Eric was diagnosed with ALS in 1993 at the age of 59, and he lived with the disease for over 25 years, passing away at 85 due to complications from a stroke and heart attack, so it wasn't even the ALS that killed him. He outlived the diagnosis of death by quite a long time. It is believed that his extensive research and adaptation of holistic treatments, including detoxification, organic nutrition, and keeping a positive attitude, contributed to his extended survival.

> Now, medical professionals are acknowledging that the quality of our lifestyle choices are determining much of our health outcomes.

Cheryl was actually on the right track when she had us go through the protocol of getting rid of sugar, organic eating, looking at everything including no microwaving foods, using only cast iron pots and pans and non-coated cookware, using filtered water, and all the things that are being encouraged in the wellness community today. That was not the protocol 15 years ago. Today, some doctors and researchers encourage us to maintain healthy metabolism and cells by carefully choosing what we eat. Now, medical professionals are acknowledging that the quality of our lifestyle choices is determining much of our health outcomes. Dr. Casey Means, M.D., has published a book, *Good Energy: The Surprising Connection Between Metabolism and Limitless Health,* that is excellent at teaching us how to eat, what to eat, when to eat, how to move, and when to move.

I don't know if doctors have come around to this way of thinking in the treatment of ALS, but I encourage anyone dealing with an illness, whether terminal or not, to seek out alternative treatments, listen to your body, and pay attention to that brain-gut connection. It is there. It is strong. It is viable. It is real.

Thank you, Eric, for your persistence, and thank you, Cheryl, for being ahead of your time as it relates to health and wellness and the holistic approach to the body.

John and I decided we would not be going back to Mayo for their ALS Clinic. At least not for a while. It was exhausting, debilitating, and depressing. There was nothing there. The only thing they could do was measure John's breathing. We would sit in a room for 6 to 8 hours while the team came and went for various lengths of time to introduce themselves, give an overview of what they provided, and tell us how they would provide it. There were no bathroom breaks, and no chance to get out for lunch, and it was excruciating and brutal for the patient. Then, to deal with the psychological implications is more than a lot of people can handle. Definitely more than people should have to handle. We talked with several individuals who did the same thing. They said, don't go until you absolutely have to. What I'm counseling is that there are resources in place that you cannot access unless you go to the clinic and get doctor's orders. So, if for no other reason, go and get the orders in place so you can access the resources available sooner rather than later. Let me say the process of caregiving is overwhelming, especially for someone like me who never thought they would be a caregiver for anyone other than their kids.

We decided on the University of Minnesota instead.

Is it surprising that Cheryl was doing her physical rehab practice when Mrs. Gonda walked in? Cheryl met Mr. Gonda through his wife who had hip surgery. Cheryl indicated that John was a patient at Mayo with a less-than-thrilling experience at the clinic. Mrs. Gonda wanted to know if we had been referred to the alternative therapies division. Who knew?

To learn that Mayo has a center for alternative treatments. Did anybody talk to us about any kind of alternative therapies, alternative treatments, alternative anything? No. They said, "He has two to five years. Go home, have a glass of wine, and get your things in order." Really?

Mr. Gonda asked Cheryl if I would mind writing a few thoughts, which I did, and those notes were sent to him. I didn't keep a copy of the notes, and I can't remember what they were about. I guess that Mr. Gonda wanted information about the level of care being provided and what it looks like for a patient who has to go through a process at Gonda. It had nothing to do with the ability of Mayo but was more about bedside manner at the ALS clinic.

John and Jeff

After returning home from the desert, John still had to negotiate his severance package with his company. Don, the company president, had fired John and left it up to Jeff, who inherited the position John had, to figure out all the details. At this point, nobody other than close family knew about John's illness, and he had been negotiating for several things within his severance package. One was the key-man policy that most companies had on their C-level executives. It's a life insurance policy Don had taken out on John should anything happen to him while he worked for them. John wanted that policy to be gifted to me. He would pay the premiums, but he wanted me to be the beneficiary of the policy.

Jeff and John were like brothers. Brothers who didn't trust each other, who fought all the time, and who didn't get along. There was rivalry, they tried to be friends. Jeff adored our boys. We did some things with them socially and tried to make it work; it just didn't.

Jeff was a man who was making the company a lot of money. His business practices were questionable at best sometimes, and John was in the division that had to make a lot of hard calls. Consequently, it was left up to Jeff to negotiate the severance, and he didn't know anything about John's condition. Well, John did tell Don he had ALS when he was let go, but Don didn't know what that was. It went in one ear and out the other, which was not uncommon for Don. So, Jeff and John went back and forth in the negotiations. John always gave Jeff the benefit of the doubt. He didn't believe in throwing people under the bus.

In February 2009, Jeff called John and invited him to meet for a drink and discuss the severance. When John told me, I got this look on my face like, REALLY? John was still fragile, and I was protective, but I said, "All right, if you need to go, then go." As soon as he left, I was on my knees, praying.

"God, please protect John and give him your peace. Keep him calm. Keep his heart open. Open Jeff's heart. Work, Lord, and may your peace and protection cover them both. May Jeff do the right thing and John do the right thing."

I prayed while I put the kids to bed. I prayed while I waited for John to come home. Several hours later, when he walked through the door, I asked him how the meeting went. He said, "It went well," and I answered, "That's good. What happened?"

He said as he and Jeff sat together, they were doing the dance of questions and answers. Jeff kept asking, "You want this life insurance policy? Why do you want it? We've worked out almost everything else. Why do you want this life insurance policy?" John answered, "Okay, Jeff, I'm going to tell you something that you've probably never heard of before. It's going to sound weird and nobody else is aware of this, although I did tell Don the day he let me go. I want this policy for Rachel and the kids because I have been diagnosed with this disease called ALS, Lou Gehrig's disease."

Jeff, who was a tough nut to crack, turned as white as a ghost as all the color drained from him. He had tears in his eyes and said, "I know exactly what you're talking about. My father passed away from ALS." They cried together. In that moment, Jeff went from being the biggest adversary to the biggest advocate for John. When he told me, I knew it was the Holy Spirit saying, *"I'm here. I'm here."* This man who had needled John for so many years and who had caused such chaos, for the two of them to be at this place in life, was nothing short of a miracle. Jeff said, "I know. I was going to quit my job and take care of my dad. I know exactly what this disease is all about." And with that, the life insurance policy issue was worked out. Amazing.

Jeff did everything he possibly could, and he checked on John in the months to come. I never saw Jeff again. I think he came to the celebration of life service, but I didn't see him. I still know today in my heart of hearts that John made an impact on him in a way that nobody else ever could. I know that when he thinks about John, he knows he did all he could. And I don't doubt there are times he might regret that he didn't handle things better, but he's okay. It was an amazing revelation. That's our God. And it's all good.

Consulting at RUSH Enterprises

The same month, John received a call from his good friend and former boss from Peterbilt Corporate, Jim Thor. Jim left Peterbilt years earlier to join RUSH Enterprises in San Antonio, Texas. RUSH Enterprises operates the largest network of commercial vehicle dealerships in North America, including Peterbilt trucks, among other brands, with more than 150 locations and 7,000 employees.

Jim asked, "Why don't you come to San Antonio? Come down for a visit. I'd like to talk to you." I told John, "He's going to offer you a job. I just know he's going to offer you a job." John replied, "I can't take a job." I asked, "Why don't you just go down there and see what he has to say?" At this point, John was still mobile, still talking, still walking. He could travel; he was slow; but he was still able to do things.

John went to meet with Jim and called me that evening. "Yeah, Jim wants me to do some work for him. He wants me to be a consultant with RUSH working on a new green project." This was terrific because John still had so much to offer.

I am grateful he was able to work until the very end. It kept him going. He worked from home, which was a new frontier for the two of us. I never had a problem officing out of the house, but now, John was having to adjust to being in the house all the time and I had to adjust to the same. Thankfully, he could still do things for himself. The consulting work was part of what got him up in the morning and kept him focused, and it went well. It's also a great testimony to Jim and the RUSH organization to hire John in this capacity.

Jim and John went to his last trade show event in Louisville that year while he could still walk and travel alone. People could tell something was wrong, though many didn't know what it was. It was bittersweet for John to be with the people he had grown up with in the business world. Eventually, everyone within Peterbilt and in trucking across the country would learn of his diagnosis.

A Spirit of Gratitude

Our faith carried us through these days, and a spirit of gratitude is evident in my journal entries through that time. We were growing in the Lord.

When I first met John, I had a lot of biblical knowledge that had been imparted to me and my siblings as a child. The stories in the Old and New Testaments, who Abraham, Isaac, Esau, and Jacob were. The story of the flood, Noah, and the rainbow.

> Our faith carried us through these days.

The stories about Esther and Purim, Jezebel and Ahab and their wickedness, and Pharaoh, Moses, the seven plagues, and "Let My People Go!" Every year, we watched *The Ten Commandments* starring Charlton Heston as Moses.

I loved the part where Moses saw a burning bush and as he neared it, the Lord said, "Take off your sandals, for the place you are standing is holy ground." When Moses came down from the mountain, he was transformed. Then, when God sent him up the mountain to receive the Ten Commandments, Moses met with Him as a man meets with a friend. When he came down, he was physically transformed. He realized that God was God! I AM that I AM. I knew the stories, but what about those people who didn't? John was one of those people,

John didn't have that background of biblical knowledge like I did, which sometimes intimidated him. In his mind, I wonder if he thought knowledge had something to do with his salvation. Having knowledge about Jesus is different from having a relationship with Him. The only thing we need to be saved is to know that Jesus Christ is our Savior, that He was born, and He died for our sins, and He is the Son of God. We believe in Him, and we declare Him to be our Savior. That's it. We don't have to know the stories of the Bible. We just need to know Jesus. There is no need for anyone ever to feel intimidated about not knowing the Bible or the characters and stories in the Bible. No need at all.

It's become more apparent to me as I go through life that when I'm walking and trusting and believing in God, my countenance changes and I feel differently, I may even look differently, and I certainly act differently. And that may be the reason we were going through this challenging period of time. All I could do was to thank God over and over and over for His goodness.

> There is no need for anyone ever to feel intimidated about not knowing the Bible or the characters and stories in the Bible.

There's a saying that good news travels fast and bad news travels faster. That was part of what was so predominant in my way of dealing with the situation. I knew when the bad news got out, it was going to travel fast, and I knew John and I were not prepared for it. That would take time. I sensed the Lord reminding me to fortify myself mentally, physically, and spiritually. Part of that fortification process was in reminding myself of all the good that God has done. Thanking Him daily for His provision, His goodness, and remembering, His way of working *all things out for the good for those who love Him and are called according to His purpose*; as in Romans 8:28.

Gratitude is a way of life for me, and it's interesting to see it recalled so specifically in these journal entries. Every day is a blessing, and we have no idea when our last day will be or what the circumstances of our last moments might look like.

JOURNAL ENTRY: FEBRUARY 20, 2009: THANKFULNESS

Thank you for John's trip and his safe return home. Thank you for a nice reunion with a good dinner.

Thank you for all the healing you are providing John daily. We thank you, Jesus, for your promise that you hear our prayers and want to answer them. Thank you for the prosperity parties booked and for more to come.

Thank you for providing this as an avenue by which to uplift others, financially, emotionally, and spiritually. Thank you for the support you have provided to move forward. Praise you, Lord.

Thank you for the money in our bank account. May we be good stewards, and may we believe, Lord, that you will continue to meet all our needs. Is there anything God cannot do? No.

Thank you for healing Ben. Continue to touch his body with your healing hands. Bring peace to Karen and Steve and heal his pneumonia, Father. He's such an inspiration. Strengthen him and his family. Thank you for the care he is receiving.

Thank you for Karen K's call today and our time to talk and share. Show her where she can be most effective for you, Father. Thank you that Jake thinks Hayley is a cousin. His confidence and belief are so sure. Faith, the size of a mustard seed.

Thank you for selling this house at a price that is fair and just for all.

Thank you for delivering John's severance package and thank you for my new opportunity.

Thank you for Scott and Jacque's 28th anniversary. Their friendship has been a blessing.

Thank you for your words. I'm desperate to know, hear, and be more like you. Fill me with your righteousness that I may serve your purpose faithfully.

Thank you, Lord, for your love. Bless us with a peaceful sleep.

I am thankful that my husband can pack and carry his bags. He looks like he's leaving for two months instead of two weeks. Why did he wait so long? It's 10:30 p.m., and he still isn't ready.

Lord, forgive me. Sometimes I just want to shake him. I am thankful for those working to find a cure, and yet I know that you are the mighty Healer of all. So, Lord, I'm declaring your power at work in John. No ALS here. I am thankful for angels. Show me how to serve you best, my utmost for your highest. Bless us with good rest.

Amen.

Thank you, Father, for all you have provided. Thank you for the children's service and the faith of a mustard seed. Everyone's comments were so kind and genuine.

Thank you for Heather's new position. May she serve you well. Continue to guide her.

Thank you for dinner with Rick on Tuesday night at Zillow with John and for sharing fun stories about family.

Thank you for Shrove Tuesday and the time to share with Pastor Brenda and Pastor Doug.

Thank you for Bible study, Linda's gifts, and Jenny's words.

Thank you for Paul taking the kids to waffle dinner.

Thank you for healing Chick.

Please bring healing to me and thank you for John's healing.

Thank you for Ash Wednesday for the 40 days of Lent. Let us be ever mindful of your sacrifice and your mercy.

Thank you for the gold opportunity. Show me what to do with it. Please help me be obedient to your will, not mine.

Thank you for John's meeting with Don today. Thank you for providing John with strength and confidence. I will continue to ask for blessings for Don and Jeff. Talk to me about talking to Don. I want to hear you.

Thank you for the gifted teachers who are committed to our kids. Continue to bless their work and prosper them.

Thank you for safe travel for John Sr., Jan, Weesie, and Tami.

Thank you for lunch with Lauri. Her insight makes me think.

Thank you for dreams. Help me and John recall them. Speak to us through them.

Thank you for a cure for ALS.

With love and gratitude, thank you for restful and renewed sleep. Amen.

These journal entries reveal that a spirit of gratitude was prevalent. I was praying things into being, calling them out as I wanted them to be, which was an exercise some spiritual teachers were suggesting.

Calling into being a cure for ALS, calling into being John's healing from ALS, calling into being travel that hadn't happened, but asking for it to be safe. It's all about the intention with which we pray and ask God for these things.

My intention was pure. I surrounded myself with teachers and believers who practiced that protocol. And so that is what I focused on.

Consulting at RUSH in San Antonio

In March, John started consulting at RUSH in San Antonio. Travel was involved, so we made arrangements that his carry-on was light, he traveled first class, and since he had a disability, if he needed a wheelchair, special seating, or whatever, he could be accommodated.

He was staying in a hotel room with handicapped accessibility. It took him longer to get ready and to do things, but he was managing okay. When he was in San Antonio, Jim was looking out for him. The boys just thought their dad had gotten another job.

John and I discussed leaving Minnesota. We didn't know exactly where we would go. We considered Dallas and California. As we were looking at the pros and cons of moving to California, the pros were that we would be close to Elaine and Van. We would have access to the doctors in Los Angeles. We would have both the mountains for skiing and the ocean for boating. The cons: more expensive housing, the political and economic climate, no lacrosse for J3, and we would be away from friends, so there would be no established support system,

We had the pros and the cons of moving to Dallas. The pros were we knew the area. The cost of living was more affordable. We had friends living there. It was easy to get in and out because of DFW, and it was a central location in the country. It would be easier to relocate Paula. The cons: we would be away from John's family, and we would have to travel to California. I thought since our story started in Dallas, it would make sense for it to end there. Besides, I had supportive girlfriends there. We set our sights on Dallas.

We decided to put the house on the market, so we engaged a realtor from our neighborhood, Diana Davis. It was a lovely home in a great neighborhood in a nice area. It was well-maintained and sat on a quiet cul-de-sac on the top of a small hill. It was beautiful. It was 2009 and the housing market had just tanked because sweeping investigations uncovered proof that millions of loans were made to people who couldn't afford their homes.

Foreclosure was the name of the game. Property values sank so low that a huge percentage of properties were underwater. We still didn't think we would have a problem selling the house.

Our goal was to be in Dallas before the next school year started. We went through the pricing and competitive analysis, and we staged the house which meant I had to pack things that might be considered clutter, clear the closets, and move stuff into the basement. That was staging number one.

When Diana's listing agreement expired, we engaged a good friend, Tonya DuBois, even though she wasn't from our neighborhood and didn't list many houses in our market. Now came staging number two. Tonya's best friend, Marcia Dolphin, was an expert in clearing clutter and staging homes, so at her direction, a storage unit was rented. We spent an unbelievable amount of money trying to sell the house. Containers were delivered to the house and furniture, bookcases, and everything we didn't need was moved into storage. We had to pack away anything personal like family pictures, personal objects, collectibles, and books because the buyer needed to "see themselves living in the home". This was staging number two.

The realtors would send a notice of each showing which had to be approved by the homeowner, who would then run around putting things in place, throwing things into the washing machine, and dishwasher, grabbing papers, and stuffing them into the drawer to hide the clutter. We got good at living a "staged" life. I don't think the second listing lasted even 90 days. John's health was declining. Getting him in and out of the house for showings was getting more and more difficult, and we decided to take the house off the market.

One thing we had not considered was staying in Minnesota, which is what ended up happening. Staying in our home was God ordained because we further developed our church community, school community, and social community, which became our support group. Girlfriends appeared. Casual friendships deepened and solidified. John's work community, the people within Peterbilt and RUSH Enterprises, were John's support group.

I am grateful we stayed. It took a long time to put down roots, but in the end, the community rallied around our family so wonderfully and were a blessing on so many levels. Other relationships went quiet. It's an interesting phenomenon how people we had spent so much time with went silent when they found out about John's terminal illness.

JOURNAL ENTRY:
AUGUST 1, 2009

Today I am sitting at Lake Carroll with the house completely quiet. No small feat with ten people, six being kids. It's about 9 a.m. and Morgan has left to help Olivia set up her party, and everyone is still sleeping.

Getting John here was a challenge, but isn't everything? Yet I do believe he is relaxing and finds Craig pretty easy to be with. The boys are in hog heaven. What boys don't appreciate the finer things in life: a jet ski, ski boat, fireplace outdoors, dogs, babies, girls, video games, and parents who are somewhat distracted?

John spent last week in San Antonio, which looks to become home for Nicole as she has accepted a position and committed to a two to three-year contract. Thank you, Lord, for providing her with this fantastic opportunity. Keep her strong and faithful and bring her ever closer to you.

Where does the time go? I sat through a presentation skills workshop on Thursday with Sage Presence and enjoyed it. I did learn some valuable things from Dean Hyers and Pete Machalek. Thank you, Lauri Flaquer, for providing this opportunity.

On Tuesday the fourth, I am speaking to a group of women business owners about the fear of success. I need to refine it a bit.

God is so at work in our lives. Every day we are granted is such a gift. I still have to cast out fear on a regular basis but resting in Him and depending on Him are becoming more of my standard operating procedure. Thank you, Father, for your loving kindness. Help me to pass it on.

In your precious name, Amen.

JOURNAL ENTRY: SEPTEMBER 18, 2009

I really must get disciplined about writing. It's good for my heart and soul. Let me recap the highlights from the past four to six weeks.

My visit with Mikki Lessard where I met Mimi Rose Helman was so inspiring. I had the opportunity to connect with Kim Fulcher, CEO of Compass in Hartford, and I met some of the other members of Mikki's team. Compass has vision, money, and focus. Kim knows so many people. She presents herself and the company extremely well. I've been coaching all my life. Lately, I've been participating in a biblical coaching online program and enjoying the work. I'm thinking that maybe I want to become a Christian coach. Keep leading me, Lord.

Nicole came the week before the kids went back to school and left on Labor Day. There had been some hiccups with her contract position. We had a great visit. We took the boys to the fair and within ten minutes on the first ride, got completely soaked.

We were on this water ride at the fair, and I heard, "Schneider family," and it's our neighbors, Suzy, and her sons, John and Scott at the same ride at the same time. Out of all the thousands of people at the fair that day, we ran into them. Thank you, Lord. We had a great time with them.

The boys rode the rides, ate, and had fun. We even caught the parade and Jake yelled at every mascot, car, truck, and rider that came by. Who does that sound like?

Nicole and I also spent about three hours working in the office. Her Registered Dietitian status let us order all of our vitamins at 50% off retail... That's a big savings.

We also looked at Compass, and she brought up some great points about certain pieces of the program, coaches, and curriculum. Then I took her to Eric's website to show her about him since I had given her the book, and lo and behold, he had just returned from Germany where he had a stem cell procedure.

I had received some info about stem cell diversification and saw this about Eric, so I jumped on the clinic site and started reading. I filled out the contact info. Nicole started checking airfares, conversion rates, and schedules.

The boys stayed out on the boat that night. She had a 7 a.m. flight, so I got her to the airport at 6 a.m. that Monday.

We prayed together and had some great conversations. All I know is that God has restored the relationship, and all of us are thankful for that.

Looking for alternative treatments was important, and God was surrounding me with people who were faith-filled, supportive and had ideas and information that might help. With each new thing we heard and learned, my hope was pushed further toward expecting a miracle. God still works miracles, right?

CHAPTER

7

STEPPING OUTSIDE THE BOX

JOURNAL ENTRY:
OCTOBER 20, 2009

It's been a month. Why is touching base here so difficult for me? It really doesn't have to be. I know I need to keep track of the "aha" moments, confirmations, and affirmations of God's amazing work in my life and in John's life. They are happening daily with amazing and divine timing. Thank you, Lord, for continuing to show yourself to us.

The XCell-Center in Germany was the next place I researched. I went online, got their information, talked to a patient coordinator, and decided we might need to take the trip. Their procedure consisted of using the patient's stem cells. Yet, I knew that the travel, the trip, and the procedure of extraction and then injecting again, would be a lot. The procedure without airfare and accommodations was around $20K. We decided to move forward and schedule a time to go; the date scheduled for the treatment was November 2.

Then, we decided not to go to Germany, but to wait and see Dr. Bigelsen, in Nevada City, CA. He was referred by Weesie's cousins, Lisa and Greg. Their daughter, Jenna, had Lyme disease for over six years. They took her to India for two months for stem cell therapy, which Lisa said gave Jenna's immune system back to her. She had been taking over 1,000 pills each week. In January of this year, she was in a wheelchair, having difficulty holding her head up or opening a water bottle. After seeing Dr. B., she started taking oral stem cells from baby pigs, which replaced most of her medication. She did a hula hoop for me in the front yard and had a wheelchair ramp-burning ceremony two days before we arrived. They are believers and I know God sent them to me so I could take John to this doctor.

Would you believe I called to make the appointment and was given the same date we were originally set for Germany, November 2? I know God has something big planned for November 2. We will be with Dr. B. for a week.

It's been rough with Paula, with whom I've had difficulties. Her dad passed away on the 17th. She left yesterday and will be gone for at least three weeks. I've been upset with her for a while due to her comment about being "the hired help." That hurt, probably more than I realized. She has pulled away from our family and, naturally, it's all my fault. I would not let her off the hook regarding not calling me about her dad, but that doesn't matter. I cried and then apologized. She was set like stone, and I left exhausted and still not feeling connected. I'm not sure if this relationship is supposed to be restored. Maybe God wants us to let go of one another, and maybe this is how we are supposed to go through it.

I am asking for direction and guidance every step of the way. God, I'm laying this before you and asking for complete and total restoration, if that is Your will for this relationship.

Alternative Treatments
Stem Cells and Grass Valley

I knew John would want to exhaust every possibility. He was analytical, logical, and he did things with a plan. There was always a plan. Yet, after we received his diagnosis, the plan changed. We didn't jeopardize our kid's future, we didn't risk anything we couldn't afford, but we made sure we did everything possible so that, at the end of his journey, we would have no regrets. We stepped into everything with the attitude, "Let's check this out. Let's see where we can go and what else we can do."

When we first received the diagnosis, we explored alternative treatments; like detox, supplements, and ionization oxygen therapy. We heard about stem cell treatment, but we felt it was too early to make that decision, so we investigated and tried other things.

I called and spoke with Dr. B. and asked if he had worked

with ALS patients, and he had not. He was honest about that, but he did believe there might be some benefit for John. He was a delightful man over the phone. We made our appointment to spend a full week in Grass Valley, CA because John needed time for his body to assimilate, adjust, relax, and process. We flew out, drove up to Grass Valley, stayed in a hotel, and proceeded to go through the therapies.

The doctor's emphasis was on the blood, which he looked at to determine what was going on inside the body. He believed the body tells a story of everything that has ever happened to us, and those things are held within the cells and the blood. He's an accredited doctor. He was also on the front lines of experimental processes so, of course, the medical community didn't look favorably upon him.

During the five days, Dr. B. gave us about two months worth of treatments. A lot of craniosacral work, an oxygen chamber, injection of animal stem cells into different parts of John's body, and then of course an extensive history of all the trauma that John's body might have or sustained throughout his lifetime. I appreciated the holistic approach that Dr. B. took. I appreciated his candor. I appreciated his time teaching us about what he was doing and showing us what it looked like in the cells, what he was seeing, and what the blood was telling him. His book, *Holographic Blood: A New Dimension in Medicine* further outlined his methodology. We had a good experience with him.

Dr. B. sent us home with fetal pig cells. John would continue to inject himself daily with the formulas given for a specified period of time. We would then sample his blood and send off a slide. This process started in November of 2009. It was after having the experience with animal stem cells that we started to investigate other options.

After our time in Grass Valley, Cheryl sent information about another doctor who did stem cell treatments. Dr. Radar used fetal stem cells for the treatment of all kinds of illnesses. The only thing I struggled with was the faith perspective of using embryonic stem cells because I've never condoned abortion. It's a tragedy that it happens yet women are going to make that decision, regardless, and legislation will not be able to stop it. I just had to believe that I wasn't adding to the underground economy of growing the abortion movement. We made the best of a bad situation, and my parents never questioned me from a faith perspective. This was my struggle and one I had to wrestle with on my own.

John and I continued praying for God's guidance.

Lord, show us how to do this because we don't know.
Lead us, tell us, guide us, just show us how to do this.

We investigated getting on board with a stem cell trial at Emory University outside of Atlanta, which would take an act of God. But to fit into their criteria, we had to agree that we may get the drug, or we may get the placebo. I understood the protocol, the things they had to do, the tests they had to run. But we were dealing with a terminal illness, and the trial was an ongoing issue with research for ALS. We didn't have that kind of time.

Lord, show us how to do this because we don't know.

Lead us, tell us, guide us, just show us how to do this.

Having the ability to gather information and make our own choices was powerful. In that power, we found comfort and peace because of the ability to make a choice. People choose differently.

In the end, we decided to give it a try. There was nothing else available, and we could afford it. We were not jeopardizing the future of our boys, and we were not putting ourselves in debt.

We did an internet search on Dr. Radar, who performed the procedure and saw the good, the bad, and the ugly. We got all kinds of perspectives and viewpoints. It was up to us to figure it out and to be discerning in making the decision that was right for us.

Making the Decision

After two or three months of praying and researching, I realized it didn't matter that we didn't know how to do this. That's why we have Jesus. That's why we have faith. He will take care of the "how." We just need to be available to Him.

We had a call with a gentleman whose son had experienced amazing results with Dr. Radar. He had a brain injury and had suffered neurological damage, paralysis, and seizures. They had seen amazing improvements in their son, who had been receiving treatments since age seven, and was now in his teens.

Dr. Radar was always available to answer questions. We asked him if he had ever worked with anybody with ALS. He had said yes, and he put us in touch with a gal whose mom had two treatments. She told us how it had slowed down the progression for her mom and how she believed it made quite a difference. Through this process, I have learned that hearing from others who have made this walk and taken this journey is so important. Whether or not I agree with the choices they made, I do respect them for choosing to live their life the way they have.

Dr. Radar was not inexpensive, and he couldn't do anything in the U.S. The two options were to go to Mexico or Dominican

Republic. He held clinics in each location one weekend out of the month. The patient made their own travel plans. The clinic was professional and organized, and everything was handled very well.

The first treatment was $20K, and anything subsequent to that was around $12K. When John and I talked about the cost, I said, "What else could we possibly spend our money on? John, we're in a position where we can afford it and we know there are trials being held with stem cells."

We knew we had to go out of the country to get this experimental procedure. We realized this was on the cutting edge of medicine. There were doctors doing trials with embryonic stem cells. We made the decision.

I had a conversation with my mom, who thought Dr. Radar might be a shyster and it might be a scam. I said,

> "Mom, if he is taking advantage of us and if it is a scam or he's a shyster, God will take that up with him. He and God can handle all that. We are making a choice. We are well-educated, well-informed individuals who are making this decision. We are putting ourselves in that place willingly, with the knowledge that it could work or could not work. He has seen results. Some people have benefited from this procedure. I believe that stem cells are, and will be, part of our medical treatments in the years to come. Whether or not it happens in my lifetime, I don't know, but I do believe that's where we're headed."

Though a little nervous about trying this new treatment, we were both confident that God was leading us in this direction, and wherever He was leading, we had to follow. We didn't know what the outcome would be, but we also knew that following God into the unknown often produces results that we might not understand. Perhaps our journey was not only for us but also for helping others. We were walking, or in this instance, flying, by faith.

CHAPTER

8

DESTINATION: DOMINICAN REPUBLIC

Mexico and the Dominican Republic

For the first treatment, Cheryl went with John to Mexico. He flew into Los Angeles; Cheryl picked him up and they drove to San Diego and crossed the border. John met Dr. Radar, who was very professional. The procedure was quick, and they were back at the hotel in San Diego having a cocktail after it was done. There was no downtime because stem cells were put into the spinal fluid. There was no major surgery. It was as simple and easy as getting an IV.

Six to eight weeks later, we decided to have a second treatment. This time, we would go to the Dominican Republic for the procedure and spend time together to relax. We flew into Miami, and I said, "We can't manage this. We have to have a wheelchair or a cart." He opted for a cart. We used some of John's travel awards and stayed in a lovely hotel on the concierge level. Every morning, we could have breakfast and then every evening, we could have happy hour and sit on the terrace with our cocktails and appetizers. It was lovely. We didn't leave the hotel. John was using a cane, and I didn't want him walking a lot because it was taxing for him. We went to the spa, hung out by the pool, had dinner, relaxed, and had good discussions.

We talked about Ronald and how he pursued experimental procedures with his AIDS treatment. We realized, more than ever, how brave and courageous he was in doing that. We never knew the extent of what Ronald dealt with in going through the treatment. John had a lot of respect for his little brother. That was a special moment.

When the day arrived for his procedure, a driver was sent to the hotel. During our 20-minute drive to the clinic, it occurred to me that we were in a third-world country getting a medical procedure that was outlawed in the United States. I wondered, what are we doing here? Why do we have to go to this particular place to have this done? It was ironic. Here we were, in one of the poorest places on earth, having one of the most expensive, experimental treatments ever.

> It occurred to me that we were in a third world country getting a medical procedure that was outlawed in the United States.

The clinic was a lovely villa with a wall around it and armed guards outside the door. It sat on the water and was beautiful. Security let us in, shut the gate, and we were greeted by five guys who helped John into the waiting area. It was comfortable, casual, and relaxing. It was inviting, like being in a home rather than a clinic.

John and I were taken to a bedroom on the main floor. The anesthesiologist, a local woman, came in and explained what would happen. I could tell John was nervous; he was always nervous about medical situations. When I'm nervous, I become chatty Cathy. John finally looked at me and said, "Okay, Rachel, just be quiet." I answered, "Okay." Fortunately, I had taken a book with me. It was a prayer book, so I sat and read and silently talked to God. Then Dr. Radar came in and everything went according to plan. He stayed and visited with us a bit.

While we were there, I met a couple who had come from Florida with their son from New York. The gentleman was in the first stage of Alzheimer's, and they were there for treatment to see if he could experience some benefits. So many people with different illnesses and diseases.

The third stem cell procedure was also done in the Dominican Republic and was a quick turnaround. We arrived on Friday, had the procedure on Saturday morning, and were supposed to be home on Saturday night, but we missed our connection in Dallas. We flew home the next morning. John was in a wheelchair for this trip, which was helpful, but it was still physically exhausting.

As John's health continued to decline, we found ourselves having conversations we didn't expect to have so soon in life. Topics covering things like death and dying and wills and estate planning ... and life support. We had hard conversations about his ongoing decline. Things like, "What do we do when you can't talk anymore?" "I can't watch you eat because when you are choking so much, I'm afraid for you." "What do we do when you can't breathe on your own anymore?"

Having those conversations with someone you love so much and have been with for so long doesn't get easier. Sometimes the conversations had to be put on hold because it was just too much to process all at once.

60 Minutes Report on Stem Cells

After Cheryl and John's first visit to see Dr. Radar, Scott Pelley, an investigative reporter for 60 Minutes, did a story about a gentleman who was taking money from people to do stem cell procedures in Mexico. In the report, the film footage showed the Medra website, which belonged to Dr. Radar. Cheryl saw the report and she called his office asking, "Are you taking advantage of these people? Are you taking advantage of my brother? Are you running a scam?" I was so embarrassed.

I wrote a note to Scott asking, "What would you do if it were someone in your family who received this diagnosis? Maybe you shouldn't be so quick to judge." About a year later, he did another story about the fact that stem cells are experimental and there was no proof that they worked.

The medical community had embraced the promise of stem cells, but the results hadn't materialized. Now, I just felt judged by someone who had no compassion for those who were willing to try this experimental treatment.

Pastor Greg's Encouragement

John's attitude about work didn't change, even though he was fighting for his life. I didn't understand why he had to be there so much, but I was learning to let God work this out for and with him. Travel was hard on his body, yet I didn't know how to stop it. If it were me, I suppose I would do the same thing. I would continue to go through the normal, routine day-to-day tasks for as long as I could. Not that John was in denial. I think that work was so much a part of his life and identity, he just wouldn't know what to do with himself, to keep his mind occupied, if he wasn't focused on something outside of his medical condition. Even when he was doing all he could do to investigate alternative treatments, his work was still at the forefront of his mind.

He spent a week in California seeing Dennis Colonello, a chiropractor; Dr. Payam Hakimi, an alternative medicine provider; Keiko Cronin, an acupuncturist; Ann Kowaleski, a massage therapist; and Dr. Hans Gruenn, who gave him glutathione.

He had a business meeting in Fontana, so I took a nap in the car while he worked, and then we had dinner with Elaine and Van in Ontario. His rhythm was go, go, go, go, collapse. Go, go, go, recoup. I knew it was just a matter of time before he wouldn't be able to travel anymore, so I held in my fear and frustration and let him do what he needed to do. My faith told me he was being healed, and I continued to ask God to strengthen him every day.

I went to Chicago to support a friend, and I met with Pastor Greg. He was thinking about transitioning out of the ministry. In sharing our news with him, I realized how limiting our religious beliefs can be regarding the possibilities of God. Pastor Greg is a man of God, and he is Spirit-filled. He shared two stories with me as encouragement.

The mother of his wife, IdaLynn, was suffering from Alzheimer's. IdaLynn was from a small family and her aunt wanted to take their mother to a healing service. After prayer and discussion, Greg and IdaLynn decided against it. I think it had something to do with not putting their faith in man, which I understand.

Pastor Greg took a mission trip to Africa the previous year. He was asked by the pastor of the congregation to pray for an especially sick child, which Pastor Greg did, in his usual way. He didn't think a lot about it because he had never felt gifted in this area of healing. But much to his delight and amazement, he received an email three months later sharing that the child recovered. It brought him to tears.

Did he believe that God worked through him? Absolutely. Did he believe it could happen again? He wasn't sure. So, it is with a somewhat cautious approach that Christians view the possibility of God in terms of what He can do and what He wants to do for us. Nothing is impossible, and God wants us to be bold and confident and ask Him for the desires of our hearts. But if we truly trust Him, we will trust that His answers, even when they don't meet our expectations or requests, are what is best.

Pastor Greg indicated that John's healing may be on the other side of this world, and I totally got that. I chose, however, not to focus on that scenario for the time being.

While I want my sons to know, from an intellectual point of view, about prayers, commandments, creeds, and catechism, which was the focus of my religious upbringing, I also want them to experience the outright amazing joy of everyday life with Jesus. That joy was something that eluded me for the first 40 years of my life, but I didn't want my sons to have to wait for the joyous, soulful experience I had been missing. I always knew that Jesus was real, but my intimate relationship with Jesus was not something that was taught or promoted by either of the religions I grew up in. Not because my mom and dad were not believers. The Baptist box and the Lutheran box were heavily fortified, and the definitions were pretty clear. I realized I might need to look beyond those boxes when we relocated again.

I went to hear Pastor Brenda Legred speak at the Chanhassen Women's Business event. She shared her journey and the story of being snowbound in her car on a closed road for one and a half days with no cell phone. Finally, a tow truck showed up with two broad-shouldered guys who pulled her out. They handed her their card and went on their way. Brenda called the number to officially thank them for their service and was told that nobody by those names had ever worked in their office. Ever! Angels? Pastor Brenda said, "Absolutely!" When she shared this story in a sermon a few months later, you just knew that people were sitting in the pew looking for a reasonable explanation. It just couldn't be an angel. This explanation was too much to believe even coming from the pastor.

> I was a prisoner of hope.

Is it that hard to believe miracles still happen? For some people, I guess it is. I was a prisoner of hope, clinging to the promises of God, enduring through trials, ready to witness what God could do. I refused to look at our circumstances through my natural eyes. Hope held me together.

SECTION II: REFLECTIONS

Reflections: Hard Days and Finding Joy

Hard days come for all of us. Sometimes they crash in like waves, one after another, barely giving us time to catch our breath. Other times, they creep up unexpectedly, knocking the wind out of us. We don't always know when they'll come or how long they'll stay, but I do know one thing: They don't last forever.

I don't say that lightly. I've had days where the weight of life felt unbearable, where I questioned everything I thought I knew, where I begged God for answers that never seemed to come. Maybe you know that feeling: the kind of exhaustion that seeps into your bones, the kind of sorrow that makes joy feel out of reach.

But here's what I've learned: Joy is always there. Sometimes it's hiding just beneath the surface, waiting for us to scratch it free. Other times, we have to dig deep, through layers of grief and weariness, just to find a flicker of it.

I've always leaned on humor. Maybe too much. When life got hard, I learned how to laugh in its face. Sarcasm became my shield. And for a long time, it worked. But it wasn't the kind of joy that heals—it was the kind that masks.

Real joy, the kind that doesn't fade when the laughter stops, comes from one place: Jesus.

There's an acronym that says JOY. It stands for Jesus, Others, and You. I believe that with everything in me. When I shift my focus from *Why is this happening to me?* to *What does Jesus want me to learn?* something shifts. My perspective changes. The weight doesn't disappear, but it feels lighter.

The holidays have a way of magnifying our emotions. Joy

feels brighter but pain feels heavier. Some seasons wreck us in a good way, reminding us of love, warmth, and togetherness. Other seasons wreck us in the hardest way, reminding us of what we've lost, who's no longer here, or how different life turned out than we imagined.

So, if this season feels heavy, reframe it. Let go of the things you can't control and hold tight to the things you can. And if you find yourself staring at a nativity scene, feeling lost, remember this: That tiny baby in the manger was the greatest gift we were ever given.

Reflections: Journaling

If you or someone in your life is going through (or has gone through) protocols for healing, you know it can be exhausting. Journaling is just like any other habit. You have to start it, do it, and stick with it to see or feel the results. I haven't always been diligent about it and sometimes didn't feel like journaling. However, in the process of putting this book together, I am amazed that (a) I had the time to do it and (b) I had the fortitude to keep doing it.

Here's the thing. Journaling is for your eyes only. Even if you never look at it again, it's the connection between pen, paper, and brain that generates the power of release, confession, and communication with yourself, your spirit, and your soul. Start somewhere. Find a journal that works for you, a writing utensil that feels good in your hand, and just start. Write your prayers, fears, tears, joys, frustrations, platitudes, and gratitude. Write anything and everything, whether one word or one thousand words. Then put it away until the next day, or week, or month. You will figure it out – just trust the process. It works.

And when you, like me, see those words again, years later, they will remind you of the thoughts, experiences, and interactions that have imparted wisdom on your journey.

One of the ways I dealt with chaos, weariness, doubt, and fear was to journal. It helped me refocus my mind and release some of the pent-up emotions. In February 2009, I started a gratitude journal and listed things that happened each day. When I look back over the entries, I can remember how God worked and moved during that season.

Reflections: Prayer

Prayer is like building muscle. The more we pray, the stronger our prayer muscle becomes. It's how we develop our relationship with God. Prayer is how we talk with God and praying isn't supposed to be a mystery. It's like talking with a friend because He is our friend. He listens and, if we will be quiet during our prayer, we can hear Him answer us back. Sometimes He doesn't answer in the way we think He should, or in the timing we want Him to answer. But we can sure trust that He has the bigger picture in mind, and He is always working for our good.

Praying is personal. I first learned about praying by watching my parents. Before going to bed every night, we were called into their bedroom. We had a devotion and then we knelt around the bed and said our prayers. Mom would usually start, and we would each add something we were thankful for or worried about. Dad would end the prayer. We did this nightly until I was around 14 years old. Even when we were too big to be on our knees around the bed, we would have our nightly devotionals that ended in prayer. For the longest time, being on my knees was the only way for me to pray. It is a position of the body in supplication.

When we're on our knees, we lower ourselves; we take a posture of humility and we submit ourselves to God, our higher power. It's an act of reverence; of deep respect.

Our prayer journey may ebb and flow. As I got older, it ebbed. I didn't pray regularly because of my busy schedule, but I always knew God was present. In the early years of my relationship with John, I don't remember praying together. Then, as we started our family, we desired to open the gates for it to flow. We both grew up in the church and were molded by the morals and behaviors of Christ, so we wanted to provide that for our children.

If you have never prayed before, it can feel weird or uncomfortable; like it's not normal. It may take time to develop this prayer practice; of having a conversation with God. Your words don't have to be fancy; you don't have to be on your knees. If we can't find our own words, we can pray the words of Jesus when He gave us the Lord's Prayer, found in Matthew 6:9-13. We can also pray the words from Psalm 23. There are many verses in the Bible that we can use as our prayer. We also have the Holy Spirit inside us who prays for us continuously, as our intercessor. He prays on our behalf and takes our worries, cares, and concerns to God, the Father. Even when we don't have the words, He does.

God hears our prayers, both big and small. He cares about every detail of our lives, so don't think He is "too busy" to be bothered with anything that is of concern to you. We need to come to Him in prayer about decisions we need to make, asking for wisdom and discernment before we make the decision. When we allow Him to direct our path, we can rest in the fact that it is His will, and He will bless it. Too many times, I've done this backward. I've made the decision and then asked Him to bless that decision; to make it okay. But that's not the way He works. He wants to be part of every detail of our life.

We can pray big prayers, little prayers, anytime prayers, all-the-time prayers, special prayers. They all matter. When I hear a siren, I pray for the person who needs their care. I pray for the drivers, the technicians, the EMTs. I ask God to give them wisdom, and that the person in need will be safe and healed. It takes less than two minutes to pray like this. Why do I pray like this? I remember being in the front seat of an ambulance when Van, my father-in-law, had a heart attack, which led to his death. I prayed all the way to the hospital. I contacted my mom and dad, who lived in Australia to pray.

So, don't get confused about prayer. Just do it. Have people pray with you and for you. You can pray out loud and you can pray quietly. You can do it anytime. Once you start, keep going and develop that prayer muscle. Pray about everything, all the time. And don't forget to stop and listen for His gentle voice and sweet promptings. And if you don't hear Him right away, that's fine. Just sit in His presence, knowing how it feels to be still and focus on Him. It's powerful but it doesn't happen overnight. But keep leaning into Him, and He will lean into you! He promises that in the Bible. (Jeremiah 29:13; Jeremiah 33:3; James 4:8)

Reflections: Don't put God in a Box. Period!

Have you ever prayed a prayer and wondered:

> WHAT now?
> WHEN will this be answered?
> HOW will it be answered?

I have. A hundred times over. Even with the faith I have, I sometimes pray, "Help me in my unbelief." In Mark 9, the father of a son with a mute spirit prayed this same thing. I know my belief is imperfect, and I need God's perfection to help me believe more.

Even though I know God's ways are better than ours: SOMETIMES I still wonder, will He be there for me AGAIN?

Because Jesus experienced life here among us, He understands these emotions and feelings. Trust is key and yet it can be so difficult. Any relationship is a two-way street, and this one is no different. He wants to hear us all the time, so don't be afraid to go to Him about the good, the bad, and the ugly. Carry on a conversation. He IS listening and, if you are paying attention, you WILL hear Him, see Him, and know Him in ways you have never imagined.

The problem is we put God in a box. Stepping outside the religious or denominational box will allow us to see what God really has to offer. I realized there was so much more to having a relationship with Jesus than head knowledge and going through the motions of what religion expects. I wanted to know more about who He is.

We want miracles. We wait for miracles. We want miracles wrapped in ways that make sense to us, answers that align with our understanding. But what if the miracle doesn't look like what we expected? What if the answer isn't what we thought we wanted? God knows the bigger picture. And when the prayers are answered differently than we imagined, it's not because He failed us, it's because He is holding us together and giving us a new hope that we didn't even know we needed. We are prisoners of hope, and it is THAT hope that carries us through.

So, if you are waiting, if you are doubting, if you are wrestling with the hard questions - keep praying. Keep talking to Him. And don't be afraid to sit in silence. Because even when you can't hear him, He Is there.

Reflections: When the Answers Don't Come

I've asked the hard questions.

> Why do good people suffer?
> Why do children get sick?
> Why does grief come so suddenly, so mercilessly?

I've sat in the dark, my heart aching, searching for some kind of logic, some kind of answer that made sense. And I couldn't find one.

There was a moment. I remember it vividly when I finally whispered, Lord, there's not even a rational strand of thought that connects all of this for me. I have no answers. I have no other option but You.

That's the thing about suffering. As much as it breaks us, as much as it shakes the very foundation of what we thought we knew, it also brings us to the end of ourselves. And at the end of us is the beginning of Him.

If you've ever been called the "spiritual one" in your family or friend group, you know what I mean. People assume you have the answers, and that your faith is unshakable. But faith isn't knowing everything. It's trusting even when you know nothing at all. It's choosing to believe that God is still good even when the world feels anything but.

Some people stop there. They know Jesus. They believe He

lived, died, and rose again. And maybe that's enough for them. But for me? I wanted more. I wanted to know Him, not just know about Him. And the more I dug into the Word, the more I realized—God isn't distant. He isn't silent. He is near.

Reflections: A Challenge for You

Tonight, before you go to bed, take one minute to pray. Just one.
If you don't have the words, borrow the Lord's Prayer.
If you don't know what to say, just whisper,
God, I'm here.
And then sit for a moment.
No pressure, no agenda.
Just be still.
I promise,
He's listening.

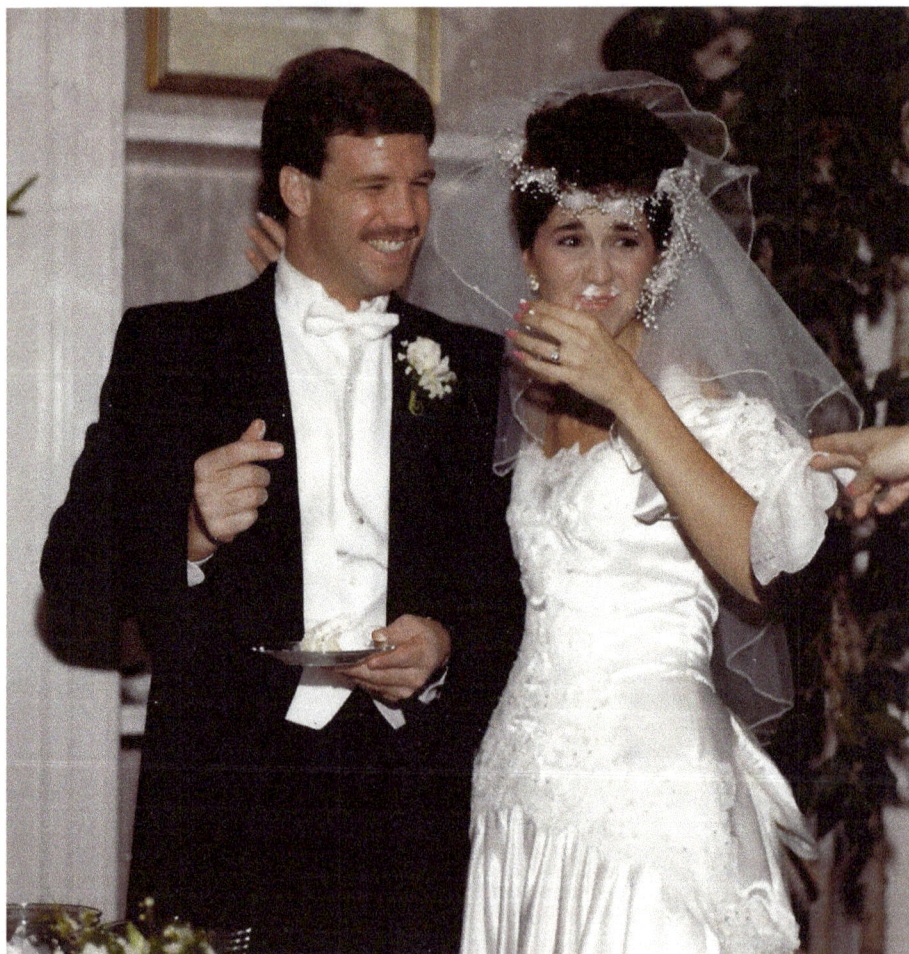

The Official Start of Our Journey Together

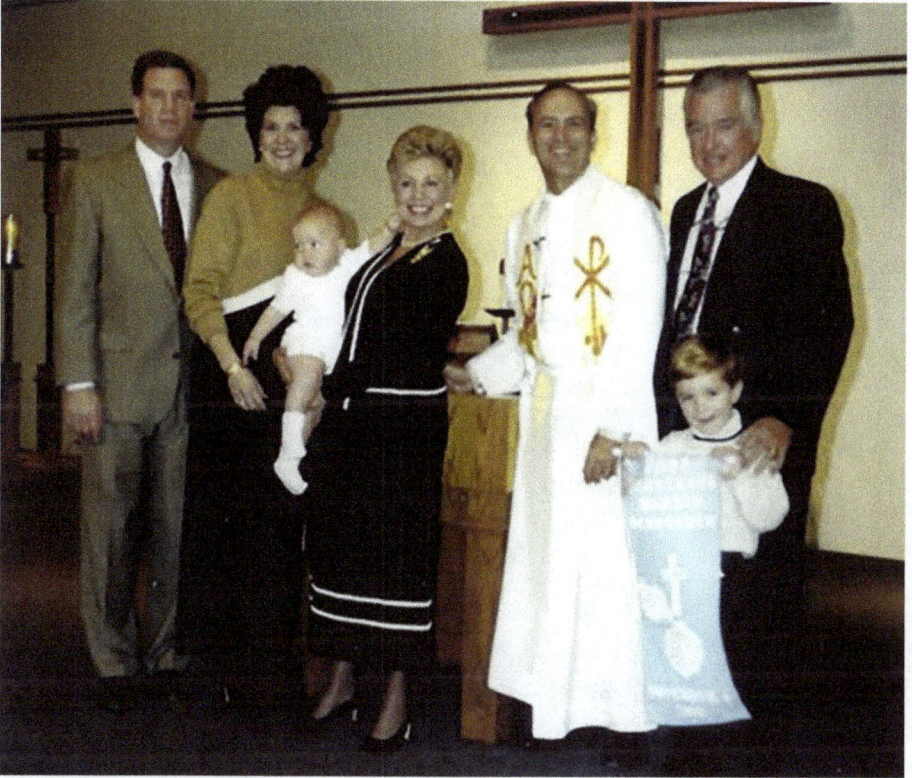

Jake's Baptism with John, Rachel, Jake,
Elaine, Pastor Greg, J3, and Van

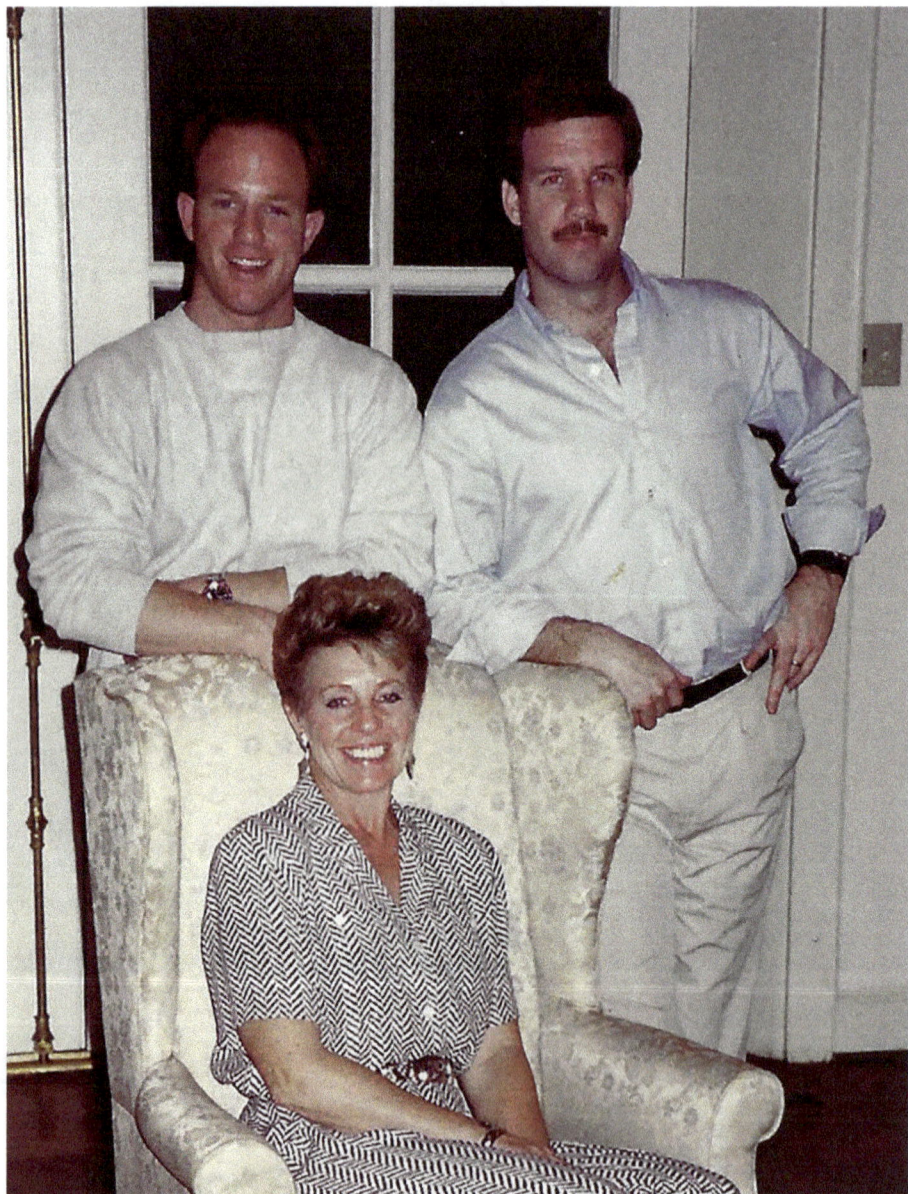

Ronald, John., and Elaine

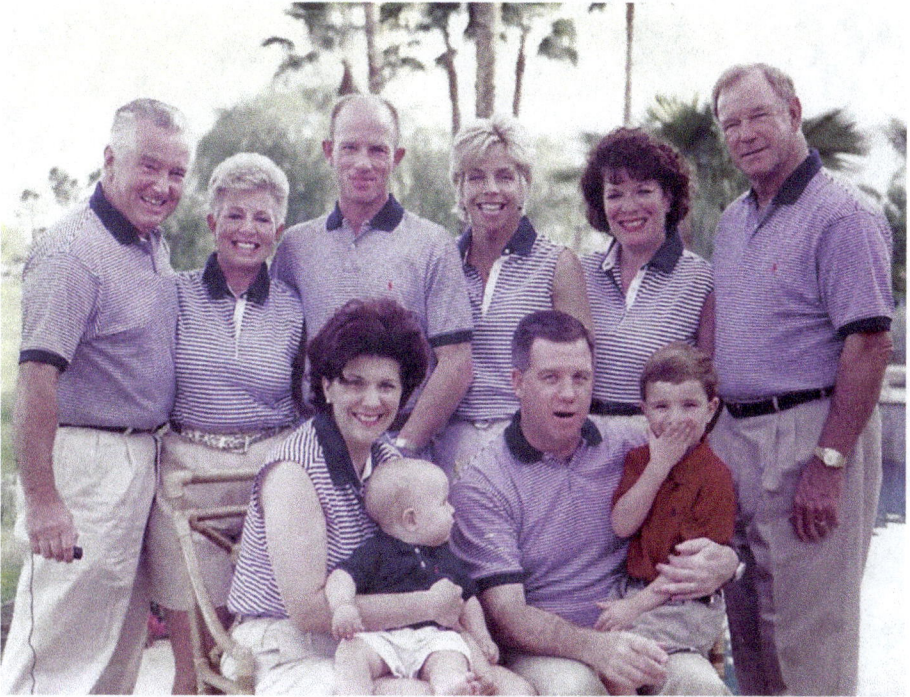

Schneider Family in Palm Desert
Back Row: Van, Elaine, Ronald, Cheryl, Jan, John Sr.
Front Row: Rachel, Jake, John, J3

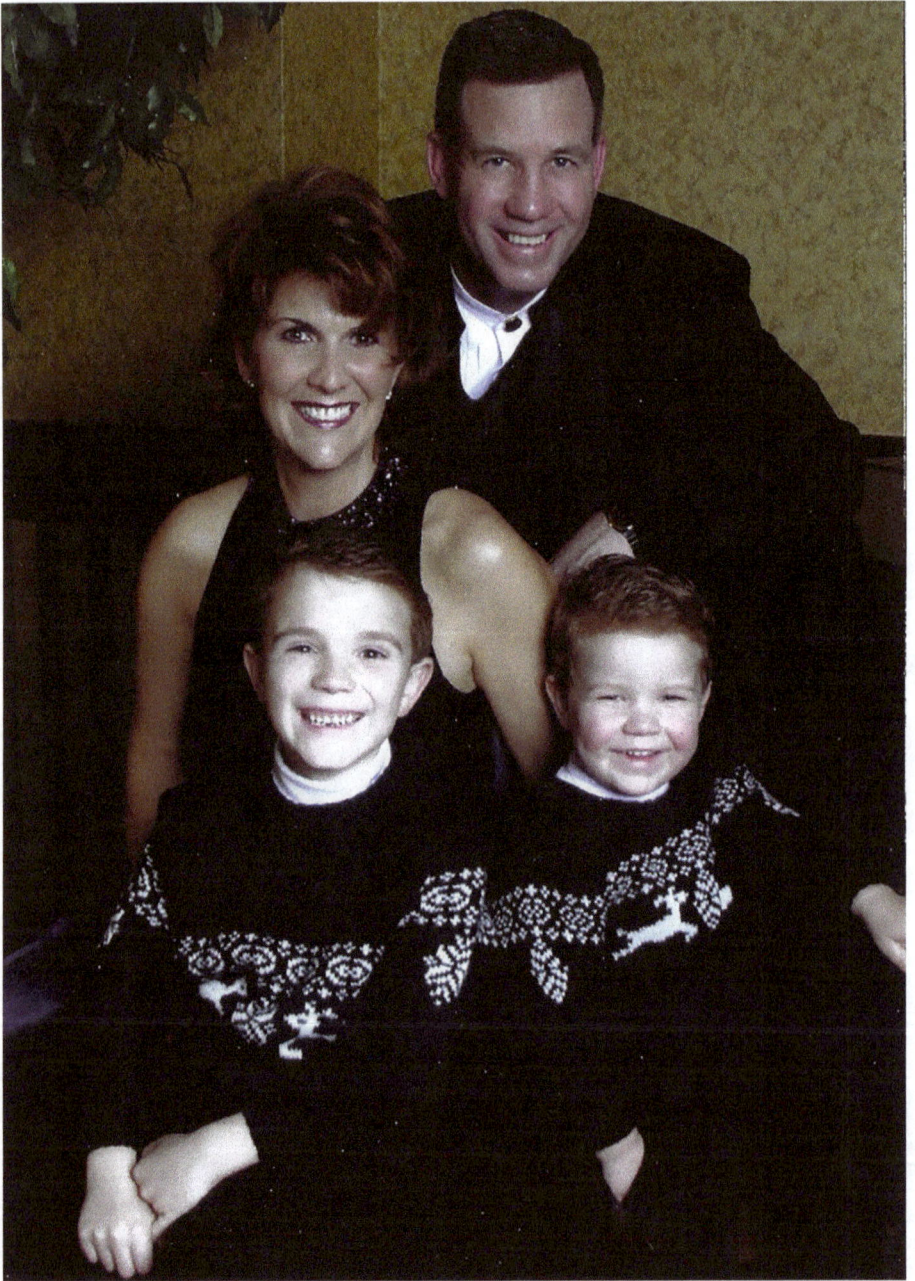

Schneider Family Portrait

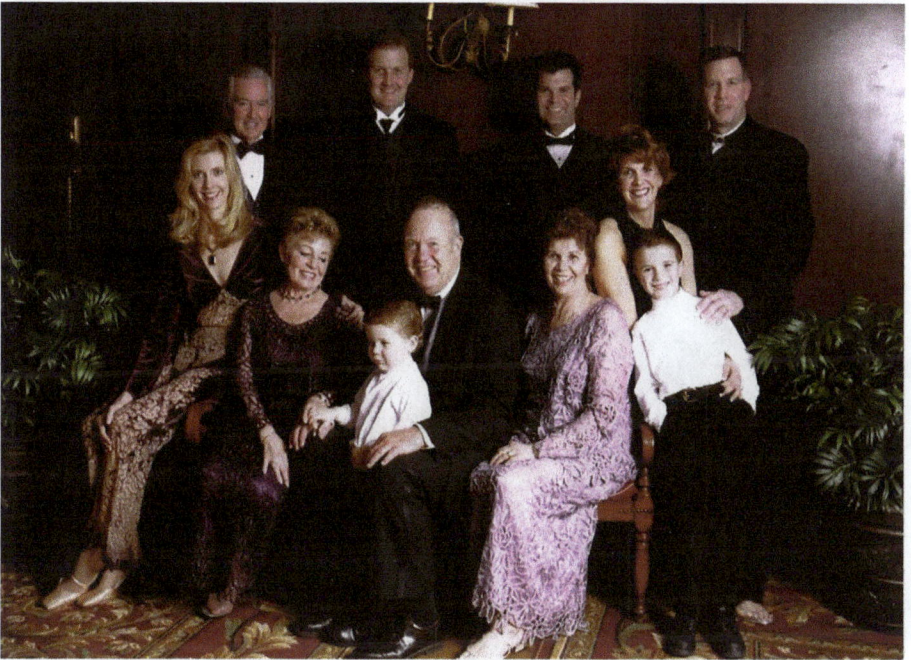

Rachel's Partylite SRVP Celebration
Back Row: Van, James III, Sean, John.
Front Row: Nicole, Elaine, Jake, James Jr., Erika, Rachel, J3

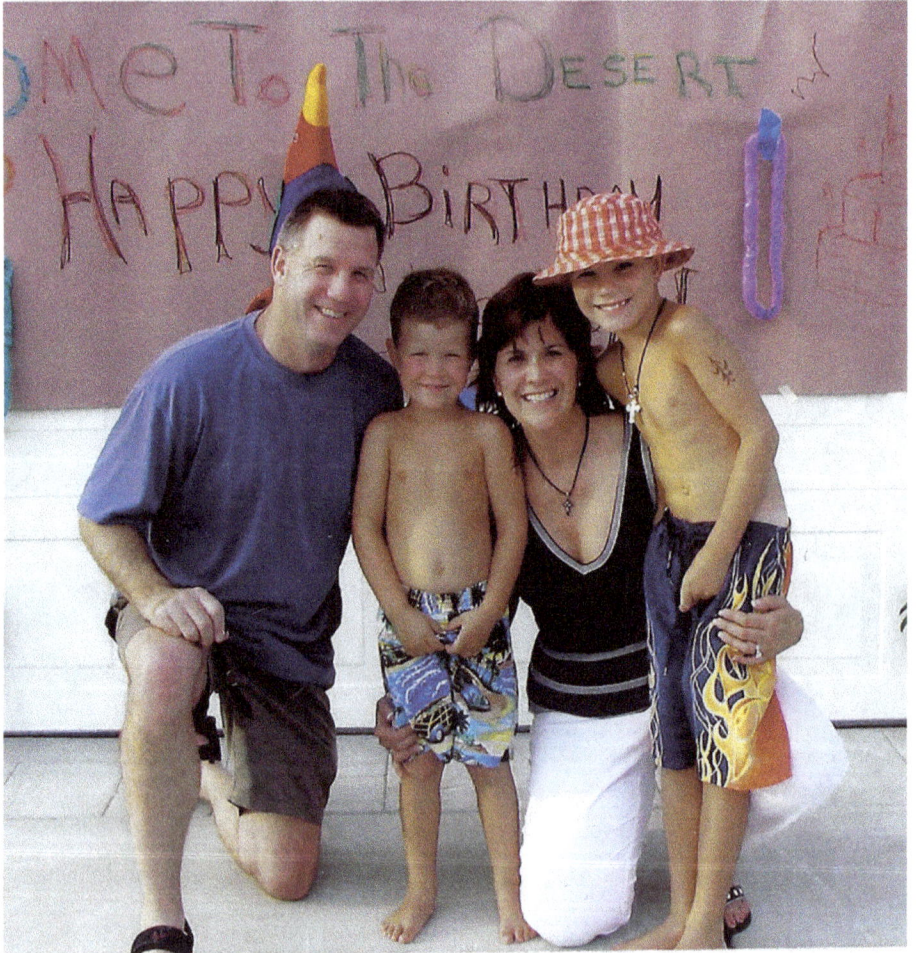

Family Fun in the Desert

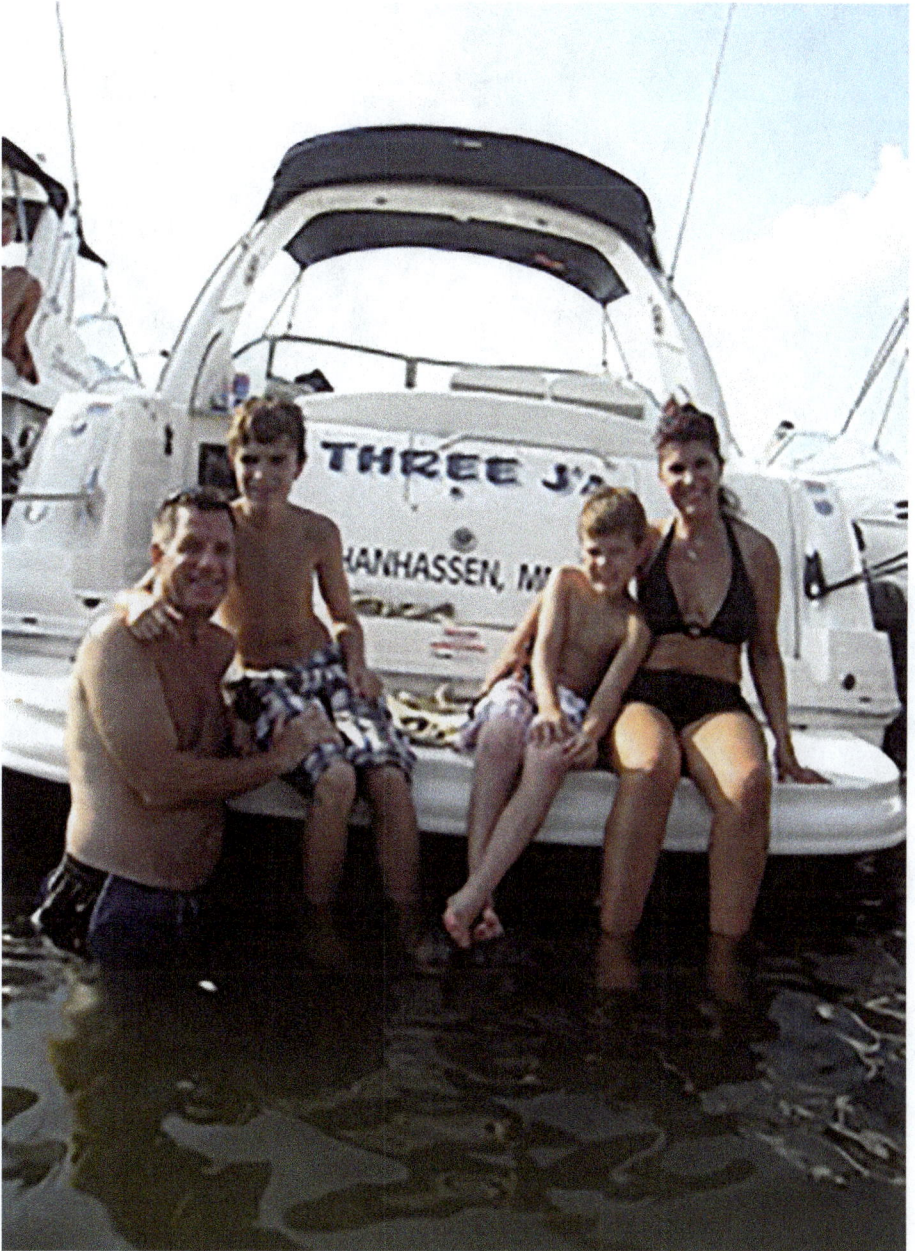

John, J3, Jake, and Rachel on Lake Minnetonka

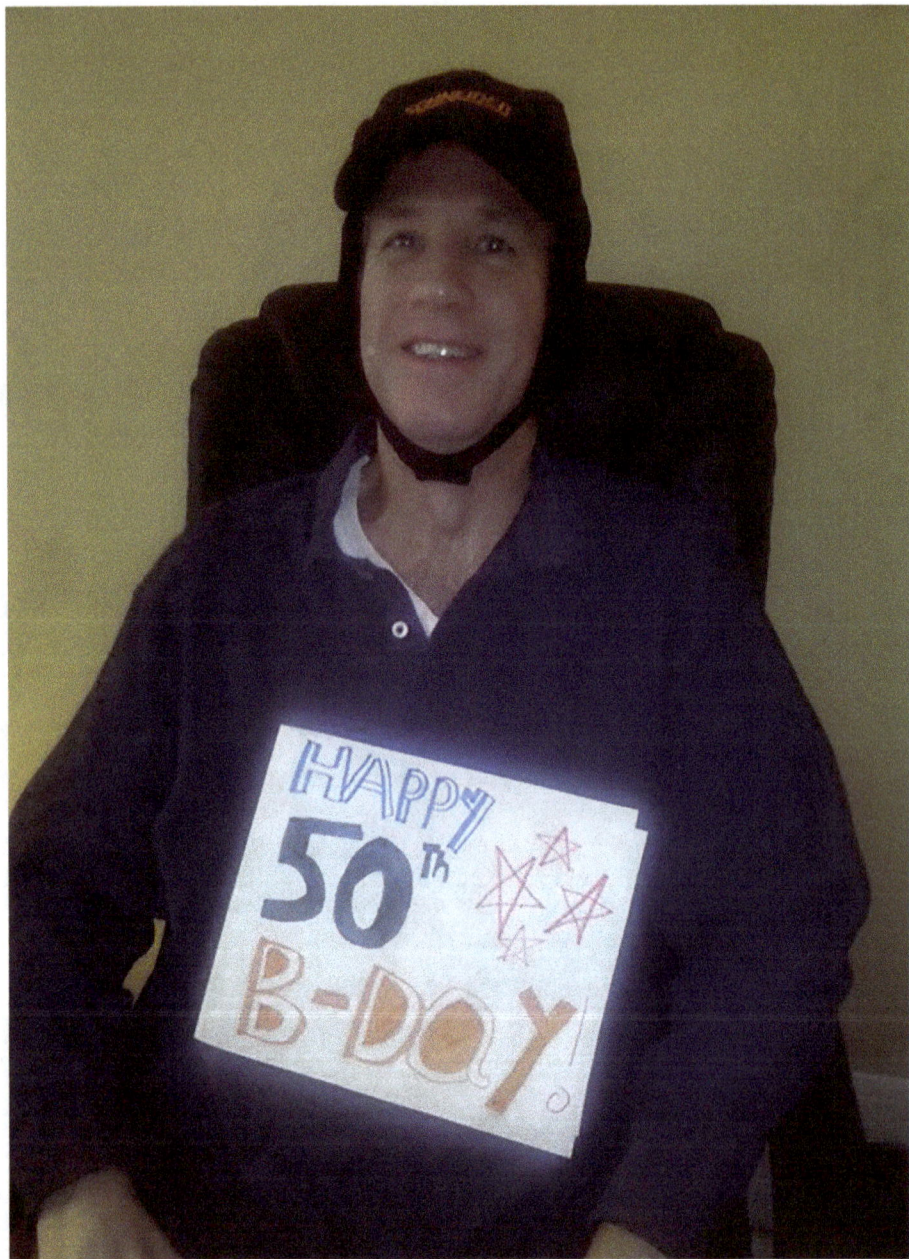

John's 50th Birthday Party

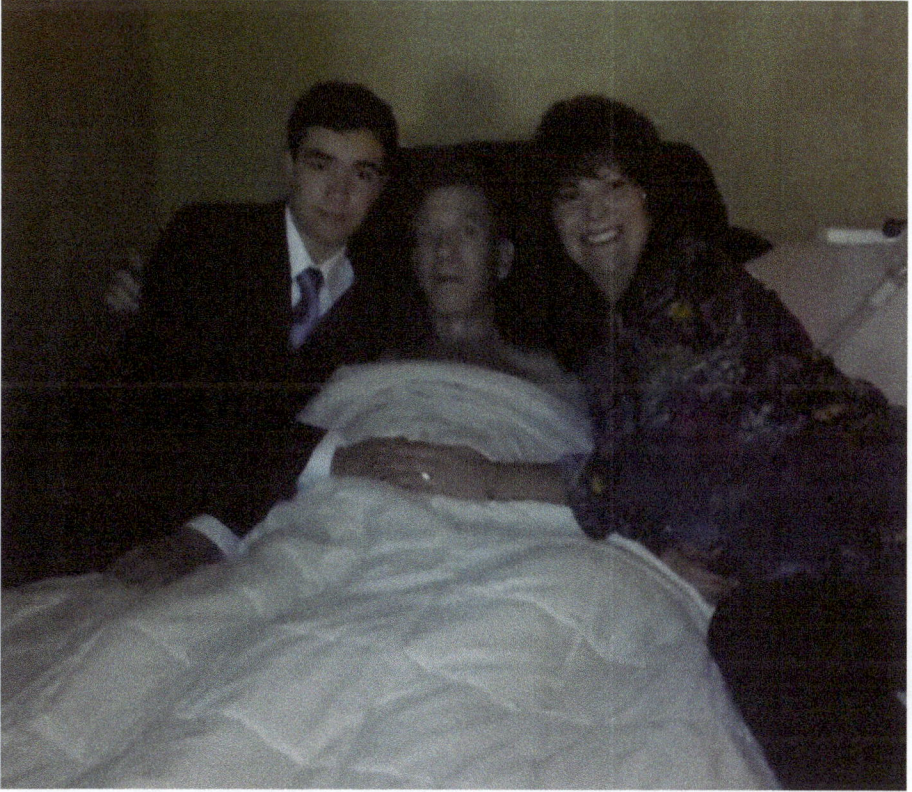

J3 Heads to Homecoming

SECTION III
BURSTING AT THE SEAMS

"As the heavens are higher than the earth,
so are my ways higher than your ways
and my thoughts than your thoughts."

ISAIAH 55:9

CHAPTER

9

GETTING IT ALL TOGETHER

Cremation Conversation

The most difficult conversation John and I had was about his end-of-life wishes. John knew I would handle everything, and he just did not want to have the conversation. There were so many decisions to be made, and he just didn't want to make any decisions, give me any suggestions, or help me figure out what his Celebration of Life service would look like. Talking about it made it too real for him, not unlike most people

First, there's the question of cremation or burial. When I was young, my family would go to the cemetery on Sundays after church and visit relatives. My dad would share his memories and we kids would meander through the headstones and then pile into the car and head home. It seemed to take forever. My mom and dad would discuss how they would one day be buried there. For them, cremation was never an option.

It's easy to see how cremation has grown in popularity. With the mobile society we live in, who stays in one place anymore? In all likelihood, my parents will not end up six feet under in Jackson, Mississippi. They live on the other side of the world, and it would cost tens of thousands of dollars to ship them there, not to mention the time, customs, and procedures. So, my thoughts were, why not speed up the process a bit, since we all end up the same way: ashes to ashes, dust to dust.

One day I went to see my therapist, Nancy, who was helping me learn to take care of myself, my boys, and John, without getting lost in the chaos of caregiving. Then I went to the cremation society of Minnesota to get information on standard cremation. I had no idea there were so many options. Urns, jewelry, decanters, charms, diamonds. I could have made John into all sorts of things. I suppose I shouldn't have been surprised. Some people just want to have something tangible to hold on to. Cheryl carried Ronald around in a ginger jar for a few years with packing tape around the lid. I felt bad for him. I didn't understand the need to haul him around.

Remember, when I first told John I needed to see a therapist, he thought I was considering leaving him. I looked at him and said, "No, honey. If I was going to leave you, it would have happened years ago. We are way past that, and I am committed to you, and us, till death do us part. And since death is going to part us sooner than later, I need to have some strategies in place to help me, you, and us, finish well. And that is exactly what Nancy and I are doing."

When I arrived home that afternoon, John was anxious about what had taken me so long. I explained that, since I was in the neighborhood, I stopped by the cremation society in Edina. He looked at me and wanted to know why. "I want to have it all done so I only have to focus on the boys when you leave us." He again looked at me like I was out of my mind. Then I asked, "Is there anything special you want to be done with your 'cremains,' as they are called?" He had no response. When I asked him if he had any special wishes about his service, he gave me a blank stare. At first, I wasn't sure he understood what I was asking. Then I realized it was just too much for him to process.

During these days, John always kept track of when I left and how long I was gone. Because of this, I was very specific in letting him know how long I would be. Looking back, I realize his anxiety heightened as he became more immobile and having me there lessened his anxiety.

Summer rolled around and of course, it was all about the boat. John and the boys did quite a few overnights at Big Island on Lake Minnetonka. The boys were good. John's foot was dropping quite a bit, and his balance was off, but for the most part, he was still good. Those times were precious for him.

John came home one weekend from one of their overnights and shared that he had told the group at Power Squadron, his boating buddies, about his diagnosis. I was shocked. How could he tell these people about his diagnosis when his sons didn't know? I said, "These guys are going to be drinking around the campfire one night and they're going to say something, and the boys are going to hear it." I was upset because I didn't consider these our closest friends. They were friends, but they would not have been anyone I would have chosen to tell first. I didn't understand that he needed to be able to talk about it. He was connected to this group, more than I was.

As it turned out, their knowing about John's illness brought him comfort. They kept his news confidential. They didn't tell our children, and it was a good thing that he shared it with them. He needed them to know.

Straight-Line Decline

The house was still on the market, and we were still showing it. We bought a new bed for the master bedroom and a Sleep Number mattress that would move and adjust. Long before he passed, in the fall of 2010, John started having difficulty getting from our bedroom to the bathroom, so he started sleeping in the guest room. It was a shorter walk to get to the boys and the bathroom, and he could "hug" the furniture and walls to make the trip. I told him I wanted us to sleep together because I would have a long time to sleep alone after he was gone. He said, "Rachel, I'm just not comfortable." I understood.

He was on a straight-line decline, and it didn't matter what we did. We couldn't hit a plateau. He was losing about 10% breathing capacity every three months, which is ultimately the demise of every person who suffers from ALS. Their lungs, actually the diaphragm, which is a muscle, stop working. With some people, it starts with their mouth and speech and their ability to eat or swallow. With other people, it starts in the limbs. It doesn't matter where it starts. It may progress quickly or not. But ultimately, in the end, they suffocate.

Telling the Boys

It became apparent that people were noticing. The boys were noticing, and John and I decided it was time to tell them. We called the boys into the family room area. They were on the sofa, and John and I were sitting on the ottoman facing them. It was around 4:00 in the afternoon. I did most of the talking. John was just too emotional, which may have been a side effect of the disease. He had developed an inability to control his emotions at that time. Anytime I had to talk to him about the boys, he became emotional.

I planned to keep it short, simple, and real. I was going to tell the truth and to answer their questions honestly. I didn't want to tell them everything as I knew that would serve no purpose except to confuse them and wear us out.

I started by telling them that Daddy was sick, and he had a disease called ALS. It was going to make Daddy's muscles stop working. It was getting harder for him to move around. They were listening. I told them that the disease was going to move through Daddy's body, and it was going to make it harder for him to move and walk and talk.

That was it. I didn't get into the death and dying thing. We didn't get into a two to five-year thing. I just left it at that because they were 8 and 12. I didn't know where J3's head was or if he was thinking, at all. Jake was the one who had three questions. The first one was, "Will Dad be in a wheelchair?" John answered, "Yes, I'll probably be in a wheelchair." Then Jake asked, "Will you ever get out of that wheelchair?" John answered, "Probably not." Then he asked, "Will Daddy get better?" I think that's when John lost it. I looked at both boys and answered, "Probably not. But what we all know is that Jesus can heal anybody of anything at any time. And we will continue to ask Jesus when we say our prayers to heal Daddy and make him better."

That was it. "Go ahead, boys. If you have any more questions or want to talk about it later, just come and let us know."

Within 20 minutes, I got a text message from Jill Johnson.

Her son, Sam, was one of the first friends J3 made when we moved into the neighborhood. Her text was, "Hey, Rachel, Sam just got a message from J3 that your husband has ALS. Is that right? Sam asked me about it." I texted her back, "Yes, it's true." She said, "OMG. I'm so sorry."

With that, the tsunami began, and John and I tried to keep our heads above water as the calls, messages, voicemails, and concern washed over us from what turned out to be one of the best community experiences we could ever have imagined. Good news travels fast. Bad news travels even faster.

I was even shocked at how soon the word had gotten out. The good news is that because we had taken the time to prepare ourselves mentally, spiritually, and emotionally, we were better able to handle the outpouring of support. It may seem surprising to a lot of people, but neither one of us fell apart when we were imparting this news to others. We were the ones that ended up providing some modicum of comfort to them. As I've stated, no doctor wants to make this diagnosis, and no patient wants to get this diagnosis. Well, no one wants to give this news, and no one wants to get this news. I don't care who you are. I wouldn't wish this on my fiercest enemy.

All these years later, the saddest thing about not having John is that they don't have their dad. Father's Day is especially hard. I hate it because they don't have their daddy. And I believe in my heart of hearts that out of everything associated with this disease, John, knowing he was going to miss watching his boys grow up was the most devastating part of leaving this world behind. He loved being a father more than anything, probably more than he loved me, and I'm okay with that.

Sip and Puff

My family has always used humor to deal with life situations, which is something I picked up and have carried all through life. This life situation clearly needed as much humor as we could pump into it.

John and I went to the respiratory therapist's office to learn how to use a new machine. Before moving him to the BiPAP, they wanted to first move him to the sip-and-puff machine. Basically, he would put a plastic tube in his mouth, take a sip, hold it, hold it, hold it, and then puff it out.

I was watching him do this and a funny image came to mind. I said, "Well, you know, my version of sip and puff would be ..." I held up my hand to simulate having a martini glass, I threw my head back and sipped down my imaginary martini. I said, "That's my idea of a sip." Using the other hand, I imitated having a cigarette and taking a puff. More like a deep satisfying drag. I said, "And that's my idea of a puff. So, when you say, 'sip and puff' to me, that's what I'm thinking." John was mortified. These were serious professionals we were dealing with, and I was cracking jokes. I thought it was hilarious.

John switched to using the BiPAP gradually as his breathing numbers declined, and he hated it, as most people do. (Many people use it to help with sleep apnea and other conditions for breathing at night.) He would pull it off in the middle of the night and just wear it for a couple of hours. Then we switched to a respirator. It still had a mask that he would have to wear. He hated it too.

CHAPTER

10

A DIFFERENT REALITY

It was Christmas 2010, and I thought we would celebrate at home. John decided he wanted to go to California. As much as this disease had changed him on the outside, he was still who he was on the inside, no matter what. He wanted to see his family for Christmas. At this point, I was letting God make our plans and praying I didn't miss a sign along the way. I was a little anxious. I knew the trip was going to take a lot out of us. He wanted it to be a really good Christmas for the kids, and maybe he knew it was going to be his last. I'm not sure that I knew.

We went to Palm Desert and stayed with his mom. He stayed in the guest room. Her house was easier to maneuver because the bathroom was a shorter distance from the bedroom. John had lost a lot of weight and was really thin. He started using a walker then. Elaine had borrowed one from a friend.

We had a nice Christmas Eve. We went to church at St. John's, like we always did. We were trying to keep things as normal as we could. We had a lovely Christmas Day dinner with John Sr. around the big table. John was eating and drinking. He looked good. He looked happy. He was wearing his red Snoopy Christmas t-shirt that he wore every year.

John's New Bedroom

On our way home from California, we were talking about the stairs. I said, "John, I don't know how you're going to get up the stairs." In our home, all the bedrooms were upstairs. It had a beautiful staircase with 18-20 steps, which were nice, wide, and fairly deep. John thought he could sit on the stairs and scoot down. But how about getting up the stairs?

I checked into an automatic chair lift that would take him up and down the stairs but found out that the staircase has to be a certain way, which ours wasn't, and then homeowners pretty much have to destroy their entire staircase to make the lift work. So, we blew up an air mattress and put it in the family room, in front of the fireplace, on the main floor. I tried to make it nice and romantic. I slept on the sofa for a couple of nights, but the air mattress was too low and uncomfortable for him.

We had to move quickly to convert the front room, which was his office, into a bedroom where he could get some sleep. Our friends came over and cleared out the office to make it his new bedroom. We situated the bed facing the window so he could see outside, look into the cul-de-sac and see the kids playing, and watch the boys coming home from school.

We put blackout curtains over the window. We put fabric sheers over the French doors so he could have some privacy. I brought in a television so he could watch TV. We brought in a chest to put some of his clothes in, and we moved a nightstand with a lamp and his BiPAP machine as well as a table into the room for when he needed to work. It was good. He was sleeping fairly well through the night, so that was good too. I bought a baby monitor so he could call me if he needed help during the night. And I thought, okay, we've got this under control.

The bed sat up a little high, which we knew would probably be an issue at some point, which happened three months later. So, we got a hospital bed. John tried it out and kept it for two nights and that was it. Out it went. He hated it and proclaimed that we were not having a hospital bed in the house. Boom. End of discussion.

Then we had the Sleep Number bed discussion. We had one in the master bedroom, and it was a good solution. I thought he would be able to move it up and down and adjust his side of the bed to make him comfortable and I could adjust mine. I said, "If you're not going to do a hospital bed, that's okay. But you're still going to need to adjust your bed. You're going to want to be able to sit up all the way or put your feet up. It only makes sense to get a sleep number down here for you." His eyes bugged out of his head as he said, "They're expensive." I agreed. They are expensive. But when someone has a terminal condition, it skews your thinking. Their comfort becomes a primary concern. So, we went out and got one. And it worked.

Making John comfortable was no easy task, and trying to find a good pillow was even harder. I can't even tell you how many pillows we went through during John's illness. Besides knocking yourself out on drugs, a comfortable pillow is the way to go. At one point we had 18 pillows that had been used at different intervals to make him comfortable.

At this time, John was still fairly mobile, he could sit and stand, although he was using a walker. He wasn't bedridden yet.

John was not a believer in sleep, or rest, or naps, and he wasn't a really deep sleeper. It only took one wrong move to ruin his night's sleep, and then he couldn't get comfortable again. I was nervous about sleeping next to him for fear of disturbing him in the middle of the night. We stopped sleeping together well before he died. And that made me sad.

I didn't realize how much not sleeping with him was going to affect me later. I knew I would eventually have to get used to it, so I told myself I might as well go ahead and start getting used to it now. I accepted it as reality, thinking it would make things better for me and for him. I had the baby monitor so I could hear him if he needed me. He could press the button and talk. But the baby monitor only lasted for two months. Then the ALS association suggested a bell (like a doorbell) that would ring if he moved his arm against it. We stayed with that bell for quite a while.

We knew we were setting up the room where he would pass. When we realized we could keep him home and that the house would work, after having it on the market for two years, we looked at each other and said, "We're done. We don't need to deal with this. This is something we can control. God wants us to stay here. There's no need to put ourselves through this anymore." We took the house off the market.

The Supernatural, Mysterious, Love of God

In January 2011, my girlfriend, Weesie, turned 50. She invited 15 of us to her lake house at Lake Leon, which we lovingly called "The W," which is about three hours outside of Dallas. Nicole drove up from San Antonio to be with us. I knew she was coming. The big surprise for me was that my girlfriend, Denise, flew in from Chicago. I didn't know she was coming. Mikki was there and Mimi Rose from the Boston area came. Lauri was there from Minnesota, and Jennifer Koch and Mary Ferrara from Texas came. And Chris Parker and her mom flew in from California. It was quite the gathering.

It was also a bit of an intervention. The care for John was intensifying. I didn't know what lay ahead, but caring for John, the boys, and everything associated with family life was getting to be too much. My girlfriends encouraged me to call my parents and take them up on their offer to come. I needed them. I needed to tell them, "It's time, and you need to get here sooner rather than later."

So, I placed a call to Australia. When Dad answered, I said, "This is the call. The call you've been waiting for." He asked, "What call?" I answered, "The 'I need you call.' Your eldest daughter is saying, 'Okay, it's time." Mom asked, "Do you need us right away?" I answered, "No, I don't need you here tomorrow, but I need you to make arrangements to get here, or at least to start getting here. And sooner rather than later would be appreciated." Dad said, "Well, we have a few things we need to wrap up or get into place before we get there, but I think we can make it by April." It was hard for me to make that call. Caught off guard by his response, I said, "Well, I'm glad this wasn't a 911 emergency call. Let me know when you've boarded the plane."

One of the lessons I was learning was to receive what people could give. The other lesson was to have boundaries on what kind of help they were going to give. But that's for later.

The Blue Orb Story

One cloudy afternoon, most of the girls decided to go into town and shop, but Nicole and I stayed back to take a walk. We walked around the lake, found a pier, and sat for a while. Nicole listened as I talked about reaching out to our parents and asking for assistance. We speculated on what the next few months might look like and how much help I would need.

We were sitting, looking into the water, and talking when out of nowhere, we saw a beautiful blue orb in the water. It is highly unusual since Lake Leon is a muddy lake, not a beautiful clear lake. I thought maybe it could be a jellyfish, or maybe it was some kind of trash that floated to the surface. It was the most beautiful intense shade of blue and it was moving, pulsing like a heartbeat.

We looked closely and there was nothing to make the orb move. There were no boats, kayaks, canoes, paddle boards, etc. So, Nicole and I sat there and watched this brilliant blue orb. I had a wonderful, warm, peaceful sensation. I was calm, tranquil, quiet, aware, intrigued, and transformed. I realized this might be supernatural, so I looked at Nicole and asked, "Do you see that?" She answered, "Yes, I do." I asked, "What do you think it is?" She answered, "I don't know."

We watched and watched and watched, and I kept thinking that, at any minute, it would disappear. It didn't. I sensed the Holy Spirit inside calm me in a way I hadn't felt before. I knew that water was important on several levels: Jesus was baptized in water. The Holy Spirit descended in the sign of a dove above water when Jesus was baptized. Water signals a new birth or rebirth. Jesus called His first disciples when they were fishing on the water. After His resurrection, He returned to them at the Sea of Galilee. And my husband, John, had a love of being on the water with the boat. It took me about 15 minutes to realize God was giving me a sign that everything was going to be okay. This shade of blue had a depth, a resonance, an intensity and an aura within it; the aura was not around it; it was in it. It wasn't glowing, but it had a light within. So we kept looking at it and talking to God, asking for His wisdom and guidance and peace and mercy. We tried to photograph it with our phone, but the image couldn't be captured; I'm so glad Nicole was there to witness it with me. After about 45 minutes, it went away. It didn't trail back out to the lake; it didn't go sideways; it didn't go under the pier. It just evaporated. Nicole and I sat there for a few more moments, letting the gravity and beauty of that moment envelope us. It connected us to our spirit and to God in a way that had never before happened. I may never experience anything like that again, but in that moment, the Holy Spirit stirred new hope within me. It strengthened and encouraged me and imparted the grace to continue.

Challenges, Birthdays, Accepting Help

John turned 50 on January 27, 2011. We marked the occasion by having a nice dinner at home. Cheryl was there and the boys were all into it. They made signs and had fun tricking out John's walker with streamers and a bell. We had a simple dinner with a beautifully set table. John was still able to eat, albeit very slowly. He was doing fairly well. It was a simple, sensational, and special birthday with cake and just a few gifts. I don't know if any of us were aware this would be his last birthday.

As John's health declined, we had people in and out of the house to check on us and offer whatever help they could. But I was overwhelmed with assistance at times. So much so that I sometimes felt as though I had been run over by a Peterbilt truck. Just because people think they are helpful doesn't mean they are and, depending on their personalities and what they like to do, they can provide help that actually makes more work. Or adds additional stress. It's interesting, too, that when people ask,

"What can I do for you?" they don't want to hear: can you wash the dishes? the windows? empty the trash? do the laundry? cut the grass? They want to do what they want to do. And depending on their relationship or connection with the one they are "helping," it varies.

In our home, we had a walk-in pantry. It wasn't big enough to get lost in, but a small child could possibly hide out for a while. It also gave space for someone to pause and consider the options for snacking, baking, cooking, or shopping. I thought it was fairly organized, even if it did have a few expired items on the back of the shelf. I have a pretty good memory, even when stressed, and I'm visual, so I knew where things were in the pantry (and in every other room in my home). The boys were younger then, so they would go in, get their snacks and get out. The pantry also had a door, so if things were a bit messy, the door could be closed.

For other people, the pantry, heck, my entire home, became their project. The interesting thing is that some of them would make the changes and tell me, and others would not. Some of the changes demanded notification. Others did not.

The pantry and refrigerator were the first lines of attack. Someone would go into the pantry to grab something and look for expiration dates, and whether it was one day or one year expired, out it went. In their mind, they were performing a major public service by getting rid of the expired items.

At first, I didn't notice. Then I was looking for an ingredient to cook or bake with and it wasn't where I had placed it. I would dig through the shelves, going deep and dark, only to discover it was gone. The refrigerator was much more immediate; the freezer, less so. Regardless, these individuals thought they were doing me a favor by continuously culling the contents of the kitchen.

I should have been stronger, or clearer, in letting people know that I didn't want to spend time looking for something that wasn't there. At least when I cleaned out the basement, closet, bathroom, freezer, refrigerator, and pantry, I knew what was gone and didn't waste time looking for it.

Declining Respiratory Numbers

John's respiratory numbers had been declining at the rate of 10%. In February 2011, we went to the clinic for our appointment with Dr. Day. There was no plateau in the decline and no stopping it. His lungs were getting weaker and weaker.

When Dr. Day came into the room, we said to him, "Give it to us straight." And he did. He told us John would not make it through the year. We asked, "What's going to happen?" He answered, "Is John going to get a feeding tube?"

John was still able to eat soft foods, and he wasn't having issues with choking, but it took a lot of energy to eat. He couldn't hold the fork, which frustrated him. Dr. Day said, "A feeding tube is a preventative measure or it's to prepare someone for what lies ahead." He recommended we get the feeding tube sooner rather than later.

This would require a hospital stay to have the procedure, and he wanted it done while John was still strong enough. Dr. Day explained the procedure. He said over 85% of ALS patients end up with feeding tubes at some point in their illness. Then I asked what percentage of ALS patients get a trach. He answered, "Less than 10 percent." I asked, "Why is that? Why is it so high for a feeding tube and so low for a breathing tube?" He explained matter-of-factly that it's because of the cost, the difference in care, and most importantly, a breathing tube doesn't guarantee that someone will live any longer. It's a lot of work and a loss of communication.

People choose to have trachs when perhaps the disease is progressing in a different way, or perhaps the rest of their bodies are still in great shape, meaning they can still use their hands and move around. But a trach is somewhat confining and it's a different quality of life and a different level of care.

I was overwhelmed. I had already had the tough conversation with John about having a trach and that I could not care for him in that state. I just couldn't. And I didn't want to. Had John insisted, I probably would have told him we needed to find a home for him or full-time care.

Because John was a logical thinker and a practical man, he appreciated the way Dr. Day presented things, and he responded to the facts. The doctor spent an hour and a half with us, giving us information. The next thing I knew, John was scheduled to have the procedure done the following week. That was the longest appointment with a doctor we ever experienced.

I didn't know what was coming, but I knew it wasn't good in terms of how it would affect John's physical body. If he was sitting and his head itched, he couldn't raise his arm to scratch. He couldn't blow his nose because he couldn't get the tissue to his face. He was uncomfortable in bed but couldn't roll over and adjust. And now, they would be adding a feeding tube in his stomach. I often wonder how he handled everything mentally so well for so long. At some point, they increased the dosage of Lorazepam, which is an anti-anxiety medicine.

I was surprised to learn how many people with an ALS diagnosis decide to end their lives, perhaps so they go out on their terms instead of going through the hell of this disease.

My esteem and usual high regard for John are magnified by his patient persistence in dealing with this horrible situation. I knew how much he wanted to be with the boys, to raise them and share with them. I had a sense that he wanted to be the man his family could count on, always and forever. John wanted to add his own signature to the storyline of fatherhood. I will always be sad that he was robbed of that chance.

JOURNAL ENTRY:
FEBRUARY 18, 2011

At 10:30 p.m., J3 texted and wanted to know if his dad was going to die. I told him I will wait up so we can talk about this. Yikes.

JOURNAL ENTRY:
FEBRUARY 19, 2011

J3 and I had a heartfelt talk about his daddy going to meet Jesus. Thank you, Holy Spirit. It went well and has created a different vibe in our relationship. I told him I would not lie to him and expected the same from him. I shared the stats of this disease. He realized his dad was getting weaker. I told him about the feeding tube his father was going to have. J3 was brave. He cried a little. I told him there was nothing we could do except pray and make Daddy as comfortable as we could.

Today after getting John up at 7:45 a.m., I headed for a massage at 8:30. I'll probably have to see a chiropractor or doctor since my right arm is going numb. Jake had a baseball clinic from 10 -11:30 a.m., then J3 had lacrosse at 1 p.m. Then haircuts for the boys, and a basketball game for Jake. We stopped by Blockbuster and rented a movie. After dinner, we watched a movie. John was tired so I wheeled him to bed and prayed he would sleep well. Thank you, God. Let me serve you with all that I am. Rachel.

Mikki called and said she had been avoiding me because she didn't know what to say. I'm surprised this is hard for her. Heck, it's hard on all of us. It's interesting how people handle grief and illness. John has gotten so soft, yet at dinner, he railed at Jake about gold pants for his Drew Brees presentation. Sometimes I wonder if he needs an antidepressant.

But I know it's just John, and as much as the disease has changed him on the outside, he is still who he is on the inside, no matter what.

The Feeding Tube

Elaine and Van were scheduled to come for a visit, so when I picked them up at the airport, I told them John was getting a feeding tube the following day and asked them to watch the kids.

The next day, we headed to the University of Minnesota to have the procedure done. John doesn't do well with needles and blood, and it took the nurse about six times to get the pre-op IV inserted. I was out of my mind. The muscles in his arms had just atrophied so much. They called in three people to get the IV going and finally brought in an ultrasound machine. They got it in, and then the procedure was delayed for hours. UGH!

After John was taken back for surgery, I made my way to the

chapel, which they call a meditation room. It had lovely stained glass, but no pictures of Jesus or religious symbols. Nor was there a chair, podium, literature, Bible, or anything else in the room to provide support or comfort to those who came in. What they did have was a corner with a stack of mats for people to grab, lay on the floor, and sit, kneel, or lay on as they said their prayers to their god. I remember thinking they missed the opportunity to minister to those who were there because their loved one was going through something hard.

I didn't realize U of M was a teaching hospital. Teaching hospitals operate differently. They have young interns doing all kinds of procedures and tests on the patients so they can learn by doing.

After John's major surgery to insert the feeding tube, we were taken to a semi-private room so he could have a few days to recover. One day, ten interns walked in and started questioning John and performing tests. I said, "You know what? The man has ALS. It has already been diagnosed, and we have been dealing with it for months. So, your poking and prodding and tapping and whatever else you're doing is not necessary. He is recovering from a procedure. So, I would appreciate you quietly leaving." And they did.

Another nurse entered the room pushing a cart and said, "We're going to take some blood." I responded, "No, you're not." She said, "Well, that's what is on the order," to which I replied, "Well, that's not happening. No blood needs to be drawn. He is not having any tests done. He has ALS and he just had a feeding tube inserted. So, we don't need any blood because we already know what's going on." I know my words were spirit-driven. I wasn't ugly; I wasn't yelling. I was being assertive in the fact that my husband didn't need any of this. I appreciated that they were there to learn, but they would have to learn by testing somebody else. He didn't need more testing.

For most of the first day, we were in the room by ourselves. Elaine and Van came to visit, and we all witnessed the formula being released into his system through the feeding tube. I gave him ice cubes and sips of water.

Pastor Doug visited the second day and presented a prayer shawl to John, but by this time, another young man was put into the room with John, and he was in so much pain and discomfort that he was wailing and screaming and cursing. We had little time with Pastor Doug due to the commotion going on in the bed beside us.

I left that night around 10 p.m. and was so upset I had to leave my husband in the same room as this person. I couldn't do anything about it, and John was so very brave. I was in tears the whole way home.

Because the University of Minnesota is a teaching hospital, I learned a lot. I learned how treatment is administered, but it mostly taught me about myself. There, I found my voice and learned to advocate for my husband. It wasn't easy to stand up and say, "Enough is enough," but I did it.

I didn't see the doctor in charge of John's case until the day he was discharged. The entire ordeal was a traumatic experience for both of us.

If you end up at a teaching hospital, or any hospital, I encourage you to push back when you don't think something is in your or your loved one's best interest. Don't be afraid to ask questions and get the answers you need to proceed. Don't be shy about speaking up. It's your right to know what's going on and it's your obligation to be heard. After all, medical treatment is not to be taken lightly. This is serious business, and someone's life or death may be in your hands. Be brave, be bold, and whatever you do, be heard.

Home Health and Hospice

In May, hospice orders were written, and we acted on them toward the end of that month. John was officially in hospice. We were told that changing the feeding tube at home could be relatively pain-free. I was nervous about it because there was a hole in John's stomach, and I didn't trust myself to know how to do this right.

We had a nurse come into the house to take care of this for us, but we didn't know her level of skill, and we didn't trust her after her first attempt didn't work. She came back and tried to fix it, which also didn't work.

Which is why in late June, John had to return to the hospital. This time we didn't go to the University of Minnesota, but we went to Fairview in Edina because they were the jurisdiction handling hospice. We had to order an ambulance and schedule the procedure. It was a process. We were trying to conserve every bit of energy we had for the important things, like taking care of the kids and ourselves. Having to spend energy on something that should have been done for us was more of a burden on everyone. I was not happy, and I let them know. Someone gave me a tip that I could change hospice organizations, and that's exactly what I did. I interviewed several agencies, which took a lot of time, but it turned out well.

Our new hospice nurse was Jim, who was a kick, and exactly what we needed. He was an angel on earth, and I am thankful we were able to make the switch.

As for home health, John was sleeping downstairs, and I was upstairs. I would put him to bed between 10:30 and 11 p.m. We had a great routine. John enjoyed listening to a beautiful George Winston piano solo album, "Autumn." The compositions were beautiful, and it calmed him. We would hear the music and start to unwind. I would tuck him in and get him comfortable, which often took a little while. He normally started on his left side, with pillows between his legs, and knees, and we would adjust the bed to lift him a little. Then we made sure the BiPAP was on correctly. He had a bell just in case he needed it, and the room would be dark. I would rub his feet with lavender oil to help him relax, kiss him, say a prayer, and shut the doors so he could have some quiet.

I was usually in bed around 11:30 and would set my alarm to wake up at 3 a.m. I would go downstairs to move him and see if he needed anything, and then wake up around 7:30 or 8:00 a.m. I was doing most of this alone during the summer but then realized that school would be starting in the fall and my schedule would need to change. In September, I'd need to start getting up earlier for the boys and would need some help with John during the night hours. So, I started looking for home healthcare. John didn't need meds or shots because his medication went through his feeding tube.

My friend, Heather Silva, worked in senior housing, and I thought she might have resources. She gave me a few referrals. We started with one agency and went through several people, working the midnight to 6 a.m. shift. They had instructions to check on John every two hours. They would arrive at midnight and check on him at 2 a.m., 4 a.m., and 6 a.m. By 6:30 a.m., I was up and dressed and ready to take over again. We did this because the kids were going back to school, and I needed to be able to sleep.

One night, the agency sent a younger girl to stay. Around 1 a.m., the bell went off and I went downstairs to see what was happening. The lights were on in John's room. He had an accident in the bed, which never happened. This young girl was trying to move him to change the sheet, but she didn't know how. She was in a state, and I could tell she was unhappy. She had an attitude that this was beneath her and that John was some weirdo. He looked at me, and I knew. We got everything cleaned up and I went back to bed. She went back to the kitchen table. The next morning, he let me know that she had yelled and cursed at him. Of course, he couldn't

> There was a time when I wondered if I would ever be able to sleep through the night.

talk back, and that was the end of that. It took me all of a minute to call the agency and let them know we would not have anyone in the house like that ever again.

For the next care team, I would leave notes, and they would leave notes for me. I still have copies of those notes, which are so poignant.

There was a time when I wondered if I would ever be able to sleep through the night. When I was a new mom, I knew that time would come. I thought those days of waking up in the middle of the night were long gone. With John's illness, it became a habit. The good news was that I didn't have to do it for more than three months. But it was hard all the same, and it wasn't fun.

Sean Moves In

My brother Sean has always had a love of aviation, travel, and the family business, which is tough. If things had worked out differently, I'm sure we all would still be in Jackson at Yazoo Manufacturing and Lawn Mowers. That's what we grew up with. My dad is an entrepreneur, and all four of his children have a strong entrepreneurial spirit.

I am the oldest and Sean is the youngest, so I'm probably the one sibling that hasn't been involved in every aspect of his life, personal or professional. When he decided he wanted out of the family business, I told him, "If you need to get away, come stay with us. There won't be any expenses. You just come, okay?"

Sean took me up on that offer and John was kind enough to agree. We had no idea how long he would stay or his state of mind. But whether he needed rest or refuge, our place was available.

When he showed up, he was a mess. We moved him into our beautiful basement which my dad called the bunker. It had a guest room, full bath, living space, patio, Wi-Fi, and a hot tub. It was a private, quiet, wonderful spot.

Sean moved in and had everything shipped from London. One night, my sister, Nicole, called and asked, "Do you know where Sean is? I need to find him right away. We were on Skype and now I can't find him." I went to the basement, and he wasn't there. I stepped into the storage room, and there he was, breathing into a paper bag. "What's going on?" He answered, "I can't breathe." "What do you mean, you can't breathe?" Nicole was on the phone talking to me, so I told her what was happening. She said, "He's having a panic attack, Rachel. We have to calm him down and get his breathing back to normal. We need to get him in to see someone."

I asked, "What? What do you mean we need to get him in to see someone? I'm the one who's got a husband that's dying. What do you mean we've got to get him to see someone? What are you talking about? I'm not even seeing someone." She answered, "Sean has some issues with his girlfriend and he's on the edge."

I was thinking, "Okay, he's on the edge. He's my baby brother. Let me see what I can do." I called my girlfriend, Marcia, who told me about a therapist, Nancy. I called and left a message, "If you can work us in sooner or later, that would be terrific."

As soon as we could, we got Sean in to see her, which was good. He couldn't sleep or eat. The relationship with the girlfriend had gotten him whacked out. I don't know the details; I just know it had not been a healthy relationship for a while. Just because we love somebody doesn't mean they are good for us.

John and Sean started spending time together, a time they had never had before. We encouraged him and he started getting stronger. We enjoyed having him with us.

Sean stayed for three months, and we were all disappointed when he decided to go back to London for Christmas. It was time for a new season in his life and we couldn't hold him back. We did what God asked us to do. We gave him a place for rest and refuge, and we encouraged him.

The front door to our house was becoming a revolving door. It wasn't long after Sean left that both family and friends started coming to visit and staying for extended periods. I wasn't accustomed to having so many people around, and I had to lean into God even more than usual to keep my sanity. Was I up for more chaos and challenge?

CHAPTER

11

HEADING TO HEAVEN

The Trip to the Urologist

Mom and Dad arrived in April without much fanfare. Sometime in July, we visited the urologist to talk about John getting a catheter because it was just too difficult to move him to the toilet. While there, I noticed we were the youngest people in the office; but of course, we were. Most people don't develop these problems until later in life. So, we waited. The moment I saw the doctor, I imagined we were dealing with another cast member of Grey's Anatomy. The young, handsome doctors were beginning to look the same.

After we walked into the office, he asked, "What are you guys doing here?" Then he read the report and saw the ALS diagnosis. The interesting thing was that John and I were not having sex anymore in the traditional way, but we were still being intimate. Recently, when our sons went away on spring break, we were alone, and we came up with a code word for our times of intimacy, "spring break."

The urologist made it clear that once the catheter went in, we would not be able to have sex anymore. I looked at John and said, "I guess there's no more spring breaks." The doctor looked at me with a puzzled look and I explained, "That's our code word for sex." He replied, "Well, you can take the catheter out and then you can reinsert it."

I think the conversation did John in. He seemed to evaporate in front of my eyes. I answered, "Oh no, once that goes in, that's it. The End." John got his catheter, which made life a lot easier. I never saw the doctor again, and that was the end of our spring breaks.

Again, I understood the gravity of the situation, but I chose to deal with it using humor. Without being able to make heavy situations light, I would have crumbled. I bet that doctor can still recall that conversation.

Caregiver Envy

The normal term *caregiver envy* refers to a caregiver who is envious of people who don't have the responsibility of someone's life depending on them; envying the freedom others have from the demands of caregiving.

I never saw caregiving in that way. Perhaps because I did have other people in the house to help. I never felt like I was tied to John's bedside. I knew I needed to be there at special times during the day. I knew I couldn't stay away for extended periods because his anxiety level would get high. For me, caregiver envy was different.

Weesie, and her daughter, Sydney, came to Minneapolis

to help me with John, and they stayed the month of July. They slept in the upstairs guest room. Weesie had hands-on experience in caregiving because she had an elderly relative, who lived with her for many years. She knew best practices like how to do transfers and how to change bed sheets with the person still in the bed.

My *caregiver envy* happened when it became apparent that John preferred the way Weesie did things like the BiPAP machine, changing sheets, or transferring him off the bed to a chair, or whatever. At first, it was kind of a joke because they would wink at each other and tease me a little about the difference in the way she and I did things. I wanted to take in everything Weesie had to share so I could remember the "right" way to do things.

I never considered myself a caregiver, nurturing was hard for me to do, I was giving it all I had, and I knew I wasn't good at it. I needed to feel his appreciation to keep my confidence up because I doubted my capabilities. I knew I had to be on guard so that my insecurities did not impact our relationship.

Caregiving is exhausting; it is consuming. It is thankless, monotonous, and challenging. Yet, giving care is one of the most tangible ways we show someone we love them. And yet, in the monotony of daily activity and caregiving, the responsibility of care is a heavy, heavy load. Weesie did it beautifully and for that especially, I am forever grateful to her.

I am also thankful that when my good friend, Mary Anne, celebrated a milestone birthday, and wanted her girlfriends to join her. Cheryl was kind enough to come in and be with John for the week I was away. I was able to readjust my *caregiver envy* when I was able to step away for a little while and remember who I was and who I was caring for.

Schneider Sanitorium

In response to all the medical needs of the people in our home, I decided to call it the Schneider Sanitorium.

My mom had medical issues to deal with, and she and my dad knew how to drive themselves to the ER. They left the house in the middle of the night without telling me, only to notify me the next morning that they had spent most of the night at the ER trying to lower my mom's blood pressure, and my dad's, too. I was shocked and surprised.

Another time, the hospice nurse took blood pressure readings on all five of us: my mom and dad, Elaine and Van, and me, only to report that everyone except me was in the stroke zone. I strongly admonished all four of them to take their meds because I certainly didn't have time to take care of them.

I thought renaming the house was funny, yet I knew there was a lot of truth behind the humor. Isn't that usually the way it works? I made the basement the orthopedic center, since that was where my mom had fallen and broken her wrist. The main floor was our neurological center, and upstairs was the sleep disorder and psychological center. The four bedrooms were upstairs. The boys and I didn't have many sleep issues, but J3's issues were psychologically based, which were revealed later. I slept fine, too, until I didn't. My sleep issues started as John's symptoms progressed. The deck was referred to as the psychotherapy and counseling area because it provided space for private conversations. I would sit out there when it was nice, and write, talk, or read. That area was a comfort and provided relief from some of the controlled chaos inside our home, which, at times, felt completely out of control.

During John's illness, my once peaceful home—my refuge

from the outside world—felt as though Grand Central Station had invaded my most coveted solitary space. For years, I had worked hard to make our home a sanctuary of calm, a place where peace reigned even when life was busy. I prided myself on creating an environment that could handle bustling family schedules without losing its balance.

But while John's illness journey brought waves of well-meaning support, that careful balance sometimes got wonky. People, often with the best of intentions, wanted to stop by to check in, lend a hand, or offer their advice—sometimes without realizing how their presence added to the overwhelming noise already filling my days. Family, though deeply loved, were perhaps the worst culprits. Their drop-ins often came unannounced, and their opinions about how to handle things spilled out without restraint. It seemed as though everyone had a perspective on what John or I should do, and they didn't hesitate to share it.

I was grateful—truly grateful—that my home was large enough to accommodate everyone. But no matter its size, there were times when it still felt like a revolving door that kept spinning, pulling me along with it until I could barely catch my breath. Some days, I joked that I needed a spreadsheet just to keep track of the constant stream of arrivals and departures, of who was sleeping where, and of which programs or therapies were scheduled for John that week.

The sheer logistics of managing all of this were draining enough, but the emotional toll was even greater. My home, once my safe space to think, pray, and recharge, became a hub of activity that never truly quieted. I missed the stillness—the precious moments where I could sit in silence and collect myself. There were days when I'd escape to my bedroom or the farthest corner of the house, simply to grasp at a few minutes of solitude.

Yet, even in those overwhelming moments, I was reminded of the deeper reason for all the chaos: love. These people cared deeply about John and about me, and their presence, though sometimes exhausting, was rooted in genuine concern. It was a messy, imperfect kind of love, but it reminded me that none of us were walking this journey alone.

Looking back, I see those moments of chaos as a reflection of the village it takes to support someone in their darkest hours. But in the thick of it, it often felt like I was being swept up in a whirlwind I couldn't control. The challenge wasn't just navigating John's care, it was also learning how to set boundaries, protect my peace, and still hold space for the love and care of others without losing myself in the process.

John started with a regular wheelchair, which was replaced by a motorized wheelchair. We had walkers, the BiPAP machine, and the sip-and-puff machine. We had the hospital tray. In the beginning, we were able to swing John's legs over and then sit him up and transfer him from the bed into a wheelchair. It was fairly easy.

I would have to transfer him from the wheelchair to the toilet. Of course, we had to get special equipment to elevate the toilet seat so he wouldn't have to sit so low and then have trouble getting off the toilet. With all this equipment, our house looked like a medical facility, which is basically what it turned into.

Then we had a Hoyer lift brought in. It's like an IV pole attached to two wheels; off that pole is a kind of crane with a winch that drops down, connects to someone, and pulls them up. It's like a lift and move, designed to allow one person, but preferably two, to move someone out of bed into a wheelchair or a different seating arrangement. And it can be a tricky process if instructions aren't followed, or if things change for the person being cared for. Either the caregiver or patient, or both, can get injured. My response when I first saw it was, "This is never going to happen. It's not going to happen here," meaning, "I'm not going to operate that thing." Never say never.

One day in August of 2011, John and I were alone in the house. He was pretty much bedridden, but he was still a fanatic about being clean. Before his illness, he showered in the morning before work and in the evening before bed. That was his norm. Now, he was having to adjust to only three to four showers a week.

Cheryl had previously come up with the idea of turning the utility room into a portable shower area for him. It was like a camp shower. Plastic panels formed a self-enclosed area, including a floor with a self-draining mechanism. Water was sourced from the sink in the laundry room. I brought in a portable heater to keep the room warm and gathered his equipment, toiletries, and clothes. The shower didn't take long, but setting everything up and taking it down was about a two-and-a-half-hour process.

On this particular day, I had to move him from bed into the wheelchair. At this point, he was like dead weight; awkward to move, and I didn't want to hurt him. I said, "Okay, honey, I can't move you by myself, so I'm going to get the lift." He looked at me like, "I don't know about this."

I had gotten good at reading him by this time. It was almost like sign language. I could look in his eyes and read his nonverbal cues. I got the straps and put them underneath him. I cranked him up and moved him over to where the chair was. I cranked him down and unhooked the contraption I had him hooked to. It looked like an episode of *I Love Lucy*, pure Lucy! John was swinging in the air; I was looking at him thinking, "Oh well, he loved all the rides at the fair, so I'm sure he's loving this. I'm sure it's no problem at all." He was looking at me like, "Get me out of here. Get me down. I want to be back on the ground."

I was trying to maneuver it; to bring it over. But it wasn't going the right way. I thought, "Let me see if I can remember how this works. I think I'm supposed to do this. No, maybe it's the other way." He would have killed me if he could have. But I finally got it right, and there he was, sitting in the plastic wheelchair.

He looked at me like this was never going to happen again and I said, "You're absolutely right. I'm never doing this again. I feel like I've put your life in more jeopardy than it already is."

My heart was in the right place. But man. Don't ask me to deal with equipment. I am not technically oriented. The Hoyer lift went back into the living room, never to be used again.

My Dad and John

When John shared his desire to learn or hear more about God, my dad was faithful in sitting with him every day reading books from the Bible: John, Acts, Romans, and the Psalms.

In John 3, the story of Nicodemus made John curious. He had Dad read it to him a couple of different times because he just didn't get it. Nicodemus was a religious scholar. He was part of the Sanhedrin, which was the political body of Pharisees and Sadducees that made decisions and implemented the law for the Jewish people. He was esteemed in the community. But Nicodemus didn't want to risk being condemned by the religious leaders, so he met with Jesus in secret under the cover of night. Jesus told him about being born in the Spirit, "No one can see the kingdom of God unless they are born again." Nicodemus was confused and asked, "How can someone be born when they are old? Surely, they cannot enter their mother's womb a second time." Jesus explained that He was talking about a spiritual birth, not a physical birth. My dad explained to John that to be reborn in the Spirit is to make a confession of faith, which allows the Holy Spirit to come into the life of the believer.

John and Denise

In August 2011, my friend Denise came to visit from Chicago. We met years earlier through Partylite when we were both pregnant. We became friends and stayed friends, and by this time, Partylite was history for both of us.

She grew up in Louisiana and her heritage was French Cajun. Her mom taught her to cook. Her parents, Helen and Edgar, visited my parents in Australia while they were there, which shows the close connection between the two families.

Denise brought her kids, and she cooked. Of course, my mom and dad wanted her to cook. Gumbo, chicken and rice, and creole were a surefire recipe for success. The house was filled with the fragrances of sauteed vegetables, shrimp, sausage, braised chicken, and gravy. I remember John looking at me, making faces. He couldn't stand the smell. She made a roux, which is a real art form, and a fancy name for a sauce made of flour and butter that is stirred until it mixes; then she added the filé gumbo spices and magic happened. My mom's mouth would water just thinking about it. It was a sweet gesture for Denise because, with her five kids, it has always been a busy life. And who has time to cook, right?

I appreciated her being with us. John wasn't happy about the cooking, which is interesting because, for the most part, there wasn't a lot of cooking going on. Because of the neighbor's generosity, meals would mysteriously show up in the "magic cooler." I hadn't had an opportunity to understand his sensitivity to smell until that particular moment.

I mentioned John's irritation to Denise, and she walked into his room and asked, "What? You don't want me to cook? Well, I'm not going to stop cooking. You better get some fragrance going in here. Let's get the diffuser fired up."

She always gave John a hard time. He loved it. He loved her very much and adored her. She was one of my friends who would give it right back to him. He was embarrassed about letting anyone see him in those last months. I think there were so many people who would have liked to come and just love him. He resisted that. But he let Denise in and that was good.

The Last Day

In the days before John's death, I kept thinking, "At any minute, this is going to be it." Cheryl came and stayed with us. We were celebrating our 24th wedding anniversary on September 12, and I think John wanted to make it to that date as well as J3 going to Homecoming. John was on the BiPAP continuously, he was down to about 120 pounds and was so thin. He didn't sip much, so we took the BiPAP mask off his face and moistened the inside of his mouth with a swab, dipped in water.

Every time I removed that mask, I thought it might be his last breath. I wasn't terrified, I just didn't want him to be in pain, and he wasn't. I knew that. We were doing a good job of making him comfortable and he wasn't moving at all. His color wasn't terrible, he just didn't look like he was with us. He had a blank look on his face. And unless I was standing directly in front of him, taking off his mask and giving him water, he was somewhat unaware.

I knew he could see outside, and I knew he could hear. I think he just lay there, listening to the sounds of the house, whatever was going on.

John died on September 26, 2011. We were having the house repainted in hopes of selling it at some point, and the painters had already finished painting the back and side and were working on the front of the house, outside John's room.

It was Monday, the beginning of the week, and they were talking about their fun weekend. John didn't like hearing their voices, so I went outside and asked them to be quiet because John was irritated. They were considerate and did as I asked.

This was the day for John to get a shower, so the hospice aide came to help. She arrived mid-morning.

We transferred John into a plastic wheelchair that could get wet. As he was getting his shower, I furiously changed the linens on his bed and freshened up his room.

We got him back into bed, all taken care of. He couldn't speak and he kept looking at something that I couldn't see. I asked, "Are you looking at heaven?" I wasn't sure because he was so far away, and he didn't answer me; He couldn't. So, I thought maybe it was going to be another rough day.

His nurse, Jim, came in to check on John around 2 p.m. John had been resting for a while because the shower wore him out. Jim told me he noticed that John's vitals were not very strong. He said, "Well, Rachel, it's your job to just keep making him as comfortable as you can. He is in the process of actively dying." I looked at him as I asked, "Actively dying? What? I've never heard that before. What are you talking about?" He answered, "Well, this is the point where the body will start shutting down." I asked, "What does that mean?" He explained that the circulation would get more difficult, his hands and feet might start to mottle, and his kidneys might start to fail. I asked something like, "Well, is he going to have a blowout, or is something going to explode?" I had never heard this term, mottle, so I wasn't sure. "Is he going to start gasping for air?" He was on the BiPAP continuously, which was different from a ventilator. I asked, "How long can this last?" He answered, "It could be a couple of days, it could be a week, but we don't know." I was shocked and bewildered, and replied, "Okay. Well, we'll just, we'll just, we'll just wait, I guess, and see."

The boys were still at school and Jim left, and my dad was taking a nap, relaxing on the sofa. I went to check on John. He was so pale. I touched his hand, and he was cold. I got close to him and whispered his name. I touched his eyes and rubbed his forehead a little, and his eyes didn't open. I got very still. I didn't want to bother Dad because he was sleeping. So, I called my mom. "Mom, could you come in here for a minute and check on John? I don't think he's with us anymore." My mom freaked out and said, "Let's get your dad." So, she called him, "James, come in here. James, James, come in here." My dad came in and, because of his military background, he had been taught to check on the life status of a soldier by opening their eyes. So, he did. He opened John's eye, and it rolled right back. My dad knew, and I knew, that John was gone peacefully and quietly, which was what John would have wanted. He didn't create a big scene for any of us. My dad started praying and reading from the book of Romans. I asked, "Dad, what are you doing?" He answered, "We're going to..." and I completed his sentence, "Finish." So, we finished, and then he started praying.

My mind was racing as I wondered who to call first. I left Dad with John, talking, praying, and reading. I called Jim, who had been gone for about 40 minutes. He came back to the house and made it official. The time of death was around 4 p.m. I asked Jim, "What do I do next?" He called the coroner.

I went to the study to look for Dad, who was talking. I asked, "Dad, what are you doing?" He said, "Well, you know, God brought Lazarus back from the dead. Jesus raised people from the dead all the time. He can do it." I love my dad for this, I love his faith. It wasn't that I didn't believe it could happen, but I had reconciled myself a long time before that if God was going to heal someone with ALS, it might as well be John. But it didn't happen. I let him stay in there and wear himself out until he realized John wasn't going to return.

Then I thought about the boys. J3 had lacrosse practice, so he wouldn't be home for a while, and Jake had football practice. So, I called my dear friend, Suzy, whose son played football with Jake, and asked if she could get Jake from practice. I told her John had passed. She was kind, sweet, and gracious.

I looked for Cheryl, but she wasn't in the house, and I couldn't remember where she was. So, I texted her. She was at the grocery store and raced back home. She came inside and saw John, then went to tell the neighbors because she didn't want the kids to be outside if a hearse pulled up to get John's body. She didn't want there to be trauma for the neighborhood kids.

The coroner sent a regular van, and the EMTs came in. I remember moving John's body off the bed, very gently, and laying him inside the body bag on top of the gurney. He was so frail. There wasn't much to him – just skin and bones. I placed a little handkerchief on his face, kissed his forehead, and said, "Oh, you're with Jesus now." They zipped him up, wheeled him out the front door, put him in the van, and drove away. I shut the doors to the study.

After John's body left the house, obviously the entire neighborhood realized what had happened. Dinner was delivered on the doorstep into the "magic cooler", as Jake called it. The boys were 10 and 14, and I made the decision not to let them see their father after he passed. I don't regret that decision. They had seen their dad every day through the disease. They had seen him disintegrate before their eyes. And although John looked peaceful, I didn't want their final memory of him to be that.

When the boys got home around 6 p.m., we went to the basement and I said, "Your father has gone to heaven." It was Jake who asked, "You mean he died?" I answered, "Yes." And we all burst into tears. I was so sad for all of us, but more for them. I said, "Your daddy passed very peacefully, and he is gone." I told them it was okay to be sad or to be mad. I think we were all just numb.

I don't remember eating dinner. I'm not sure who I called or who Cheryl called. The boys went outside because some of their friends had gathered outside the house in the cul-de-sac, just to be available for them. The friends tossed the football and tried to engage them in activities they enjoyed, to distract them for a little while.

Then, it was time for Monday night football, which was the thing the boys did with their dad every Monday night. It had always been a great bonding time for them. The Cowboys were playing so we watched the game. Then we went to bed. I don't know how we slept, or if we slept. I just don't remember.

CHAPTER

12

THE RELIEF IN GRIEF

Celebration of Life

When I realized John would be going to heaven, I didn't want to hastily plan his Celebration of Life. I hadn't been in a hurry for three years, so why start now? And since John had been cremated and many people would need to travel in for the service, I wanted to take my time.

Naturally, John, like his brother, didn't leave any instructions or preferences. He just knew I would get it done. And, while I did, it would have been nice on some level to know what he would have wanted. A song, verse, photo, prayer. The only two things I knew for sure were that Jim Thor had been asked to speak, and Pastor Greg was to be part of the service. Beyond that, John and I didn't talk about it. Ever. Maybe he didn't want to; maybe he thought he had more time; maybe it just wasn't something he wanted to deal with. I knew he would want a party, a gathering, and with so many guests from out of town, it only made sense. I knew it had to be kid-friendly because of the boys and wanting to have their friends there.

When I look back on the planning and preparations for the celebration of life events that I hosted, I realize that my experiences in marketing and promotion allowed me to organize and produce these events so well. Even in the face of huge sorrow, this knowledge did not escape me and allowed me an outlet for my emotions. I was able to channel my energy in a positive way that resulted in events that beautifully honored both Ronald and John.

Jake was 10 years old, in fifth grade, and John was 14 and just started high school. After consulting with Pastor Dave and the calendar, we decided to have the service on Friday, October 7 at 11 a.m. followed by a pizza lunch in Luther Hall. The party was scheduled for 6:30 that night at Bayview.

I was more than willing to let a few people do what they do best: coordinate and facilitate. And they did, with flying colors, which left me time to focus on what was important: the boys and the message; the focus of the service. Pastor Dave and I spent time looking at verses and discussing format, timing, etc. I then mentioned that we would like for Pastor Greg to be part of the service in some way. I gave him a little bit of our background and left it at that. I had songs to choose and a picture to find for the program.

Fortunately, Weesie, who had moved in with us for the month of July, had already been scanning photos and we had a lot to work with. Carolyn, whose son Leo was a friend of John's, was amazing in producing a first-rate video review of John's life, as well as designing the program and the thank-you notes. She also provided her skilled services as a photographer.

During that time, the thought crossed my mind; perhaps a video could be shot of the service and perhaps later at the party. What better way to capture the essence of John than to have friends and family share their stories on film that the boys and I could review at a later time.

John certainly didn't want this much attention, not in life and certainly not in death. But at this point, there wasn't a lot he could do about it, could he? Too morbid? Not for me, especially since John had been young and left behind young sons. I wanted the boys to be able to hear about their Dad from others, not just me.

And let's be honest, I could not remember everything either. I made a call to Ryan Corcoran, who had shot videos of me for over five years with my work. He was a young, bright go-getter, and he was touched, delighted, and somewhat intrigued to add this type of project to his resume. He checked his calendar, said yes, and that was taken care of. To this day, that was one of the best decisions ever. The finished product is fun, sentimental, bittersweet, and sincere. It was what mattered most as people reflected on John's influence in their lives. One of the brightest moments was to hear Jake's friends talk about Mr. Schneider: football, food, faith; it's all fabulous.

Paula attended John's Celebration of Life. She visited with people she had known through the years of being part of our family. That was the last time I saw her. She passed away from cervical cancer several years later.

Why Wasn't it Me?

I couldn't believe it. John's death certainly wasn't anything I could have seen for myself. Yet, somewhere in the back of my mind, I wanted it to be me instead of him. Why not me? Why him?

Why the logical analytical one? The one who was so smart about everything. The one who had been so good. His mom had already lost one son. Why did she have to lose another?

I didn't understand what he was telling me when he said, "*They think I have ALS, I need you to go back with me to Mayo tomorrow while they run more tests.*" "*ALS? What are you talking about?*" That conversation felt like a million years ago. The fact was it had only been three years. And here I was, sitting in the pew, wearing a red dress and listening to people eulogize my husband.

Why red? Especially when the custom was to wear all black. Honestly, I had never thought of wearing anything other than red. Red is a color of celebration, fire, and force. I was celebrating. And I knew John was too. We were celebrating his release from pain, paralysis, and this awful disease that had consumed him. I was celebrating love, the kind that never fades. Red represents the flame of the Holy Spirit and the fire of faith that refuses to be extinguished. I always thought red was the perfect color for me to wear, and then I discovered red is the signature color of the ALS Association.

John would have been the proudest of his boys. Jake and John. For weeks, Jake had rehearsed a poem called *The Dash*. His brother chimed in a few days before, so like him, saying he wanted to say the poem too. Jake, in his generous, typical fashion, agreed. And now they were both in front of me. In front of the church, filled with 600 mourners. Our boys recited the poem and encouraged people to wear the blue wristband in memory of their dad.

I listened as my father and father-in-law spoke of John. My father fashioned himself a minister of sorts and had been dying to get behind the pulpit. John's death gave him that chance. He had written, rewritten, and rehearsed his remarks for the two weeks between John's death and his Celebration of Life. I joked that even the squirrels had grown weary of listening. I was glad that I decided to videotape the service. I knew I would always remember it. I just wanted to make certain I remembered it right. Too bad I hadn't done it for Ronald, but John would have thought it was ridiculous. He probably thinks that even now. I guessed that I might be starting a trend. I've always been just ahead of my time in a few strange ways.

As I sat listening to the family, I wondered why I hadn't decided to speak about my husband. After all, I have little fear of public speaking and was known to have a way with words every once in a while. I realize that I just didn't feel the need. It was as simple as that. Everything I needed to say to John had already been said. People either knew it by now or they didn't. Those past three years taught me so much about my faith, my family, my friends, my frustration, my fortitude, and my future. More than anything else, I learned about myself and that I would have gladly traded places with my husband.

As I looked toward the front of the church, there were two exit doors on either side of the altar; one on the far left and one on the far right, which was where the choir and pianist usually hung out. Both doors were designed as exit only, not to be opened from the outside. To exit, the door had to be physically pushed.

Near the end of the service, before we were dismissed for the reception, there was a noise that sounded like the closing of a door. At that moment, it was a reminder to me that John had been with us, witnessed, and heard. He had celebrated, worshipped, and testified through his life and his death to his family, his boys, his friends, his colleagues, and that community. He had testified to the goodness of God. And that door opening and closing was him, leaving the building and saying, "I'm good. I'm good to go, and I am gone." And in that moment, I was made aware that he was good, in a good place, and that the boys and I would also come to rest in a good place as well.

Though I was ready to meet Jesus and leave this world, that wasn't His plan. God had more work for me than I could imagine, or maybe I couldn't. But what I knew at that moment was that John had finished well.

Reflections: Caregiving - The Unseen Weight of Love

If you're a caregiver, I see you.

I know the weight you carry: the exhaustion, the uncertainty, the moments where love and frustration tangle so tightly you can't tell where one ends and the other begins. I know how caregiving stretches you, physically and emotionally, how it presses into the deepest parts of who you are.

Maybe you're caring for an aging parent, their once strong hands now frail in yours. Maybe you're looking after a child with special needs, balancing fierce love with aching exhaustion. Maybe it's a spouse, a sibling, or a dear friend—someone you never imagined would need you in this way.

Whatever your situation, I need you to hear this: You are doing enough.

Caregiving is not about perfection. It's about presence. It's about showing up, even when you're running on empty. It's about holding on, even when resentment whispers in the quiet. And if resentment does creep in—if anger, exhaustion, or envy slip through the cracks—let me remind you: That doesn't make you a bad person. It makes you human.

One of the hardest lessons I've learned is that you are not meant to do this alone. You are allowed to ask for help. More than that, you need to.

I know what you're thinking: I don't want to burden anyone else. But what if, in asking for help, you're giving someone else a blessing? What if someone is waiting for the opportunity to step in, to serve, to love?

If you're in this season, my prayer for you is simple: that God gives you strength, patience, and a heart that keeps giving without breaking. But also, that you give yourself grace; that you rest when you need to, that you breathe when you need to, that you remember: you are not alone.

Reflections: God's Healing Power

Did we pray for John's healing?
Every day.
Did we believe God could heal him?
Without a doubt.
Did he get healed the way we wanted?
No.

John died of ALS. That was our reality. That was our heartbreak.

But does that mean God didn't move? That our prayers didn't matter? That He let us down? Absolutely not.

John was healed. He just wasn't healed here. He was healed in heaven, in the presence of Jesus, where sickness and suffering no longer exist.

It's hard to sit with that, isn't it? We want healing on our terms. We want miracles that fit our expectations. I've had so many conversations with my boys where I had to say the hardest words a mother can say:

"I don't have the answer. But Jesus does."

I still don't have the answers. And I probably never will this side of heaven. But I do know this: God's love didn't fail us. His presence never left us. His grace carried us through.

If you're in a season of unanswered prayers, I get it. I've lived it. Keep holding on. Keep asking the questions. And when the answers don't come in the way you expect, lean into the only truth that matters: God is still good.

Reflections: End-of-Life Planning & the Grace of Letting Go

If I could have traded places with John, I would have. No hesitation.

I was ready to go. I still am. Meeting Jesus doesn't scare me. But what does shake me is knowing how many people, even people of deep faith, still say they aren't ready.

I don't understand that. I really don't.

What I do understand is preparing for the inevitable. If I had been the one dying, I know exactly what I would have done. I would have written letters. I would have recorded videos. I would have made sure my children had something to hold onto long after I was gone.

I would have planned my Celebration of Life service and laid it out so there were no questions, no last-minute scrambling, no "what would she have wanted?" conversations. Not because I needed control, but because I wanted to make it easier for everyone else.

So why didn't John? Or Ron?

John was methodical. He always had a plan. But not for this. Maybe it felt too final. Maybe it was too much. Maybe it was just too soon. And I get that.

But here's what I've learned: End-of-life planning isn't about death. It's about love. It's about lifting the weight off those left behind. It's about giving your family the gift of clarity, of direction, of peace.

Because in the end, the programs, the flowers, and the printed words on a page, all fade. What remains is the way someone is remembered, the way they left their imprint on our hearts. That's the legacy. That's what matters.

And sometimes, even in grief, we need humor. We need to laugh in the face of the hard moments. We need to find light, even in the heaviness. I promise you, laughter doesn't erase the pain but it does give us room to breathe.

Reflections: My Opinion of John's Obituary

John was always matter-of-fact and would have wanted his obituary to be to the point and simple. Something like this:

> John William Edward Schneider Jr. was born in Atlanta, Georgia on January 27, 1961, to John and Elaine Schneider. He attended Lewis and Clark College where, in addition to his studies, he played football. He graduated with a degree in business and finance. His 15+ year career with Peterbilt included various sales positions. He joined W.D. Larson Companies in 2004 as president and most recently consulted with RUSH Enterprises.
>
> John is survived by his wife of 24 years, Rachel, and their two sons, John III (14) and Jake (10); his parents, his stepparents Donald Van Hoff and Jan Schneider, and his sister Cheryl Ingram. He was preceded in death by his brother Ron.

Reflections: Being an Encourager

If you find yourself in a situation with any kind of care, don't be afraid to speak up. I know it's exhausting. Whether you're caring for yourself, your parents, children, siblings, or relatives, you owe it to yourself to get the help you need.

My heart goes out to people who have to find care for their loved ones and my heart goes out to the people who have to provide it. It's just a tough spot all the way around.

Part of my role in life and what I've been called to do is to encourage. I can encourage people without having to agree with them or give them specific guidelines. I can speak my mind in a loving and gracious way. I can encourage them to be their best self and to take the time to do what they need to get themselves in that place.

Reflections: Losing Someone & The Moments That Stay

What would you do differently if you knew today was the last day for someone you love?

I've asked myself that question a thousand times.

The truth is, I didn't know John was going to die that day. The hospice nurse told me he was "actively dying," but what does that even mean? It didn't register.

Looking back, I'm grateful I didn't fully understand. Because if I had—if I had gathered everyone around his bed in some kind of death watch—that moment would have been ours. It wouldn't have been his.

Instead, he left this world the way he lived in it—in his own way, on his own terms, surrounded by love.

His passing wasn't drawn out. It wasn't full of dramatic final words or long goodbyes. It was peaceful. It was quiet. It was exactly as it was meant to be.

And that? That was a gift.

But even knowing that, some images stay.

I remember zipping up the body bag.

That's a moment you don't forget. It's one of those images that sears into your mind, one that lingers long after the rest of the world moves on.

My sister-in-law, Cheryl, said, "I can't stop seeing it."

I told her, "You might not stop seeing it immediately, but the sharpness will fade. The memory will stay, but the pain won't always feel this raw."

And I believe that.

Because grief doesn't go away, it changes. It softens. And faith blunts the sharp edges.

I haven't spent much time asking "Why John? Why us?" but I have wondered, "Why Elaine?" She watched both of her sons get weaker and succumb to their sickness. I really cannot imagine how her heart hurts at times, yet I'm probably one of the few people in her life that comes close to understanding how she might feel. Her resiliency is remarkable, and I marvel at her energy and enthusiasm for life. It's in her DNA, and it runs through all her family.

Six years after John's death, Elaine lost Van unexpectedly. She had just turned 80. It has crossed my mind more than once as to why Elaine lost both of her sons to diseases for which there is no cure. AIDS and ALS, both striking when these guys were in the prime of their life, both of them so different, yet so much alike. Losing a child is tragic. Losing another one within 10 years is horrific.

Reflections on Life After Death

People ask me, "Has John come back to you? Have you felt him? Heard from him?"

The answer?

No. But I have felt God.

One night, not long after John passed, I rolled over in bed and looked up. The ceiling was full of flames—not roaring fire, but soft, flickering blue and gold gas flames, moving in a rhythm, pulsing with life.

At first, I thought I was dreaming. But then I heard it—not out loud, but in my soul.

"John is good. You are good. I am with you. There is nothing to fear."

I felt warmth. I felt love. I felt overwhelming gratitude to the point of tears.

I didn't grab my phone. I didn't wake the boys. I just laid there, soaking it in, knowing deep in my spirit that God had never left me.

I didn't need a sign from John.

I had the presence of Jesus.

And that? That was everything.

John and Jake - The Dash

John's Celebration of Life

SECTION IV
ALL THINGS NEW

"You will go out in joy and be led forth in peace; the mountains and hills will burst into song before you, and all the trees of the field will clap their hands. Instead of the thornbush will grow the evergreen, and instead of briers the myrtle will grow. This will be for the Lord's renown, for an everlasting sign, which will not be destroyed."

ISAIAH 55:12-13

CHAPTER
13

NEW BEGINNINGS

Celebrating the Tribe

After John's death and Celebration of Life service, I wanted to find a tangible way to thank "my tribe." These were the women who had supported me daily through this life-and-death experience. Elaine had a beautiful home in the desert, Casa Grande, and I wanted to take them there as my way of showing my gratitude. So, I hosted a dinner party at my home and invited all 12 of them, with their husbands. I set an amazing table. It was at this dinner that I told the guys they were going to have to get their calendars out. They were going to be on call because their wives were not going to be available. I was taking them away for three or four days. They were all shocked. The men were like, "what?" The women were like, "what?" But for different reasons. It was so much fun; it was one of my favorite things. That dinner party was delightful. I made the plans for our trip, giving them several months to make necessary household arrangements and prepare for adventure.

Then came the remodeling and redecorating projects. The downstairs office where John died was turned into a cozy study. My fabulous books, cozy chairs and great lighting were installed. We had also turned the basement into a man cave for the guys. They had built-in shelves for sports memorabilia and things they loved. We put in a wet bar with a refrigerator, microwave, a game area complete with an electronic whack-a-mole, a console with electronic games, a dartboard, a beautiful TV area, and a sectional sofa that was also pull-out. The basement looked amazing.

Discovering Myself Again

During this time, I met Susan Bigham, who was also a new widow. Her husband, Dave, had died of a heart attack while working out. I didn't know Susan very well when that happened. One of the questions she asked was, "Where's the handbook?" She had two children to navigate through the grief and newness of being a one-parent family, and she had the same questions I was working through. I got to know her very well.

If anyone would have told me that my life could look this way, I don't think I would have believed them.

I remember having a discussion with John about my remarrying, and he could hardly talk about it because it made him so emotional. But he did want me to be happy. I was determined to be on a different trajectory. I was going to go to work. I was building a platform to inspire, empower, uplift, and encourage other women. I planned to speak at women's Bible conferences, write, and do all kinds of stuff.

When I shared my goals, John looked at me in surprise like, why would you do that? I have taken care of you financially. You don't have to do that. But I wanted to.

I did several events with the Canfield Training Group and attended multiple trainings. While I was learning a lot about myself with Jack Canfield and Patty Aubrey, and laying a solid foundation for speaking, writing, and publicity with Lauri Flaquer, this new life didn't lend itself to being a single mom with young boys. This grieving process was going to take us to places we had never been before, and I needed to spend time at home and be available to my boys.

I set my dream aside, realizing that if that was where God wanted me, that door would not close forever. So, I focused on the boys and discovered that was enough.

Children grieve differently than adults. My attention and focus needed to be on what was right in front of me, namely, J3 and Jake. And I needed to spare a bit of time for myself, too, so I continued to see my therapist. It didn't take too long before I realized my son, J3, was careening off the curb.

CHAPTER

14

LIFE AFTER JOHN

Relocation was always part of the agenda; rehab was not. And then there was the matter of my parents who were still with us. They stayed for a while and then it was time to send them back home. I decided to put the house back on the market. This was staging number three. It took a long time to sell. Staying in Minnesota during John's illness was the best decision, and I am grateful for the wisdom God had in helping us see that.

J3 needed time and space to deal with his struggles and addiction. We had to do an intervention to get him the help he needed. He went into rehab at Caron, in Wernersville, Pennsylvania at age 17.

While he was in rehab, Jake and I decided it was time to make the move back to warm weather. His dream was to play high school football, *Friday Night Lights* style. Jake reminds me of his father physically, mentally, and emotionally. I told him we would move anywhere he wanted to go. I really meant that. He had been through so much, and I really wanted to serve him. So, after much discussion and prayer, I found and bought a house online in the DFW area. Jesus is the best realtor.

I had been a pampered wife who always had corporate moves where everything was packed for me. This move was not a corporate move, so my girlfriends came and helped me pack, and we packed everything ourselves. We did it bit by bit; you don't pack up a house in a day. The movers just loaded up the furniture and the boxes and that was it. And then, the "one day" comes when it's done. The last person with me in the house was my friend Susan. She was with me as we shut the door for the last time.

We moved into our new home, our haven for happiness, on December 15, 2014, and the unpacking began. J3 was getting out of rehab for good behavior and planned to spend Christmas with us. Van and Elaine were flying in. I was anxious because I wanted it to be one of those Norman Rockwell holidays, yet there was so much to be done. It wasn't picture-perfect, but it was real and reminded us of the true spirit of the season.

A Different Life

I love Dallas. If I never live in the cold, ice, or snow ever again, I will forever sing praises to Jesus.

Every time I have moved back to Dallas, it has been different. It was good, but it was also important to realize that it was going to be different before I set myself up for major disappointment. People move on with their lives, and sometimes when they come back, if they come back, they are different.

I will never forget about John. We have a hallway in the house I call our memorial gallery. It has John's portrait with "The Dash" poem over it.

Life after John was filled with a lot of what people call the "new normal." Forget that. There is no new normal. I don't know who came up with that. It's catchy, but that's about it. Every day is a new opportunity to share our spirit, our faith, and our gifts with the world. To be part of His plan for our life. Every morning, I thank God for waking me up and letting me see another day. I ask, Lord, how can I serve you today? How can I step into what you have planned today? Because that's what I want.

SECTION IV: REFLECTIONS

Reflections: Grieving

With adults, some grieve well, and some don't. The community grieves differently. Grief is a whole new ballgame. I am convinced our culture does not do it well, but we are making progress.

Reflections: Keep Breathing

Life often brings us hard things. Unexpected things. It's interesting how these situations occur in our lives, and we don't know why. There are times we don't know how to respond or deal with them. These moments take our breath away and we forget to take another breath.

It's important to keep breathing.

It's important to talk to Jesus and to keep talking to Him.

The Holy Spirit will reveal strategies for the situations.

See a counselor if you need to.

Do the work.

Ask the Holy Spirit to help you do the work, because on our own, we're just not capable.

The change won't happen overnight but keep going. Keep pushing.

It's a great life I have now, even with everything that still gets thrown at me daily.

I'm overwhelmed by God's goodness, His faithfulness, and His promises.

And you will be too—just take a moment to reflect on all He's already brought you through and the beautiful things He still has in store.

'Being confident of this, that He who began a good work in you will carry it on to completion until the day of Christ Jesus.' — Philippians 1:6"

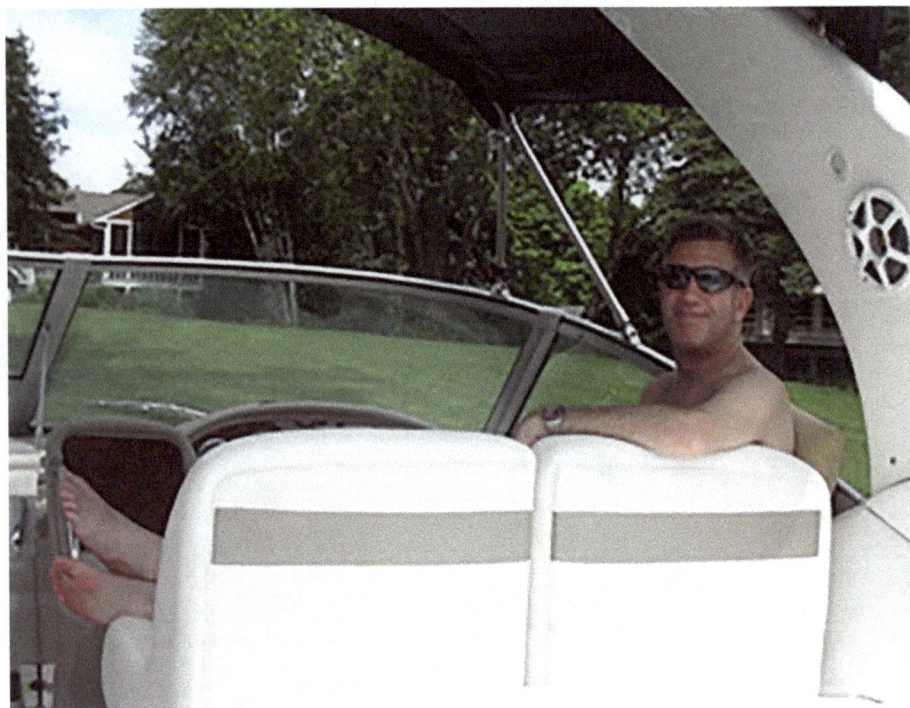

JOHN'S PRAYER

Dear Lord,
until you call me by your side...
please strengthen my heart
to be able to gently let go
of the ones I love.

As my thoughts seem to be
all I now possess,
please Lord, keep my mind clear
to praise Your love and Your protection
Without Your guidance in my life path
where would I be?

Dear Lord, please enfold my wife Rachel,
my sons Jake and John,
my mom Elaine, papa Van,
my sister Cheryl, and all those who have stayed by my side
with their presence
or with their thoughts
in Your sweet embrace;
and please help them accept
what cannot be changed,
and maintain peace in their hearts
and strength of character
to face life's hurts
as You are helping me...

Your son, John

THE STORY GOES ON…

The Boys, The Bible, and The Battles

Grief doesn't play fair; it strikes, then lingers, unraveling even the strongest of families. For John III and Jake Schneider, the death of their father to ALS at just 50 years old turned their world upside down.

At 14, J3 had just stepped into the turbulent halls of high school, grappling with the agony of loss while seeking solace in the wrong places. His charm and wit, once his greatest assets, became his shield as he spiraled deeper into a shadowy world of marijuana, harder drugs, and dangerous friendships.

Jake, at 10, took a different path. A natural athlete with boundless energy, he threw himself into sports—baseball, lacrosse, basketball, and football—anything to outrun the heartbreak and distract from the chaos unraveling at home. He was a son determined not to add more weight to his mother's already unbearable load.

For Rachel, the loss of her husband was more than just the end of a love story—it was the start of a battle to hold her family together. Juggling therapy appointments, support groups, church, and the excruciating maze of addiction treatment programs like Hazelden, she found herself stumbling, falling, and rising again, all while trying to keep her family afloat. Her faith became both her anchor and her battleground as she wrestled with questions no prayer could immediately answer. She often wondered if her resilience would continue to rise above every situation.

Through broken curfews, shattered trust, and fleeting moments of hope, *The Boys, the Bible, and The Battles* take readers on a raw, emotional journey of loss, resilience, and redemption. This poignant sequel to *The Widow Chose Red?* reveals how faith, perseverance, and unconditional love can flicker in the darkest moments—and how even when the road is rough, the heart never gives up on family.

AND IT CONTINUES⋯

God, The Guy, and The Girls

In the touching and triumphant conclusion to the trilogy, Rachel and Kevin's journey together begins. After years of navigating loss, love, and long-distance challenges, they marry and blend families. However, the lives of these children are not without complications, obstacles, and growing pains that need to be worked through and overcome. Rachel and Kevin must rely on their faith and resilience more than ever.

Without fail and through each hardship, just when they think they've found a rhythm, life throws them more unexpected curveballs: Isabella's dreams pull her to Chicago, John wrestles with a decision that could reshape his future, and Rachel and Kevin must confront a secret from Tara's past that threatens to disrupt the fragile harmony they've worked so hard to create.

This is a story of second chances, unshakable faith, and the power of love that refuses to quit, even in the face of overwhelming odds. Will Rachel and Kevin's carefully crafted plan for their family's success hold strong, or will their devotion be tested one last time?

Prepare to laugh, cry, and cheer as this blended family discovers that love and grace are always enough. Even when life feels anything but.

ABOUT THE AUTHOR

Since her husband died in 2011, Rachel's faith continues to be challenged by widowhood, single parenting, a son with an addiction, relocation, relationships...a new husband, after ten years of long-distance dating, bonus mom to four girls who lost their mom to breast cancer, and becoming a YaYa, unexpectedly.

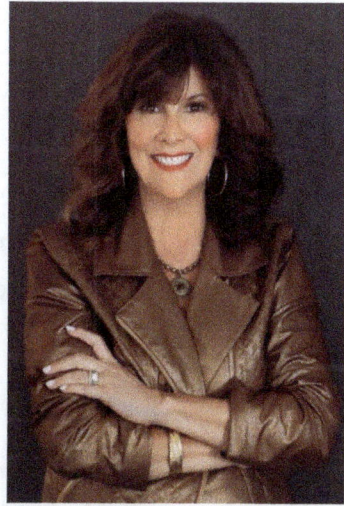

Through it all, her reliance and relationship with Jesus has given

Rachel Kerr Schneider

her the resilience that only the supernatural power of the Holy Spirit can provide. Her mission is to remind women that they do, in fact, possess a super-power of their own in the form of the Holy Spirit which lives and breathes in each one of us.

Rachel is a member of the National Association for Christian Women Entrepreneurs and BRI Talks. She enjoys travel, which is good, since her parents live in Melbourne, Australia.

She is a graduate of Cottey College and holds a B.B.A. from Southern Methodist University. A southern gal at heart, she currently calls the Dallas area home.

On a professional level, Rachel created Spirited Prosperity to provide support, encouragement, and inspiration for women seeking to grow their faith, with a special emphasis on their relationship with the Holy Spirit.

Her work has included personal training with Patty Aubrey, co-author of *Chicken Soup for the Christian Woman's Soul,* and Jack Canfield, co-creator of *Chicken Soup for the Soul* series; Ignite with Lisa Nichols; John Tesh's All Access Coaching; and Platform with Michael Hyatt.

As a Senior Regional Vice President for Partylite, she was a contributing author to the bestseller *Build It Big* and has trained and spoken with hundreds of women.

Visit Rachel's website where you will enjoy a Spirited Sentiment at www.SpiritedProsperity.com. The QR code for the website is provided below. A portion of book sales will benefit The Live Like Lou Foundation.

Rachel's Website:

Feel free to contact Rachel for speaking engagements, book signings, or to share your story of trial, resilience, and healing at info@SpiritedProsperity.com

www.ingramcontent.com/pod-product-compliance
Lightning Source LLC
Chambersburg PA
CBHW062129020426
42335CB00013B/1157